THE LOW-CARB
RESTAURANT GUIDE

THE LOW-CARB
RESTAURANT GUIDE

*Eat Well at America's Favorite
Restaurants and Stay on Your Diet*

CHERI SICARD

M. Evans and Company, Inc.
New York

M. Evans and Company, Inc.
216 East 49th Street
New York, NY 10017

Library of Congress Cataloging-in-Publication Data

Sicard, Cheri.
  The low-carb restaurant guide: eat well at America's favorite restaurants and stay on your diet / Cheri Sicard.
    p. cm.
ISBN 1-59077-062-5 (pbk.)
  1. Restaurant--United States--Guidebooks. 2. Low-carbohydrate diet.I. Title.
TX 907.2.S52 2004
647.9573--dc22

                                          2004011583

Designed and Typeset by Evan Johnston

Printed in the United States of America

0 9 8 7 6 5 4 3 2 1

Contents

The Restaurants A-Z

Introduction
Low-Carbers Unite!

Now more than ever, it's a convenient time to be on a low-carb diet. Grocery stores and restaurants throughout the country are recognizing the sheer volume of people who choose to reduce the carbohydrates—and more specifically, the *refined* carbohydrates—in their diets.

Local, regional, national, and international chain restaurants, consistently found in large cities and small towns across America (and sometimes across the world) are realizing the enormous marketing niche low-carb dieters represent. Never in the history of restaurant food have we had more choices. Low-carbers can now enjoy everything from low-carb sandwiches to lettuce-wrapped cheeseburgers to sugar-free margaritas, cheesecake, and chocolate mousse at their favorite restaurants!

It's amazing how rapidly things are changing. While researching this book, restaurants that had a small selection of low-carb items when I began are now launching full low-carb menus and marketing campaigns. Needless to say, I was changing and updating until the last minute. Undoubtedly there will be more changes after this book goes to print. Every restaurant I spoke with that had already implemented a low-carb focus to their menu has found it to be wildly successful. Even those who have yet to incorporate specific low-carb options into their menu report a staggering number of requests from customers for burgers without bread or entrées with steamed vegetables instead of potatoes, pasta, or rice.

KEEP IT UP!

The low-carb revolution is well underway and it's only

going to get better. The more vocal we—the people living the low-carb lifestyle—are, the more carb-legal foods we'll see on restaurant menus and supermarket and convenience store shelves. If you don't see something you need or want, ask for it. If store or restaurant managers get enough requests, they will try to accommodate them. Another way to encourage the growth of easily accessible low-carb foods is to patronize those stores and restaurants already offering them. Let restaurant managers know you appreciate the low-carb options and that you'd like see more of them.

Although I tried my best to compile a list of as many restaurants as possible, there were some chains that I was unable to include. For some of these, the low-carb information simply was not available, while others requested not to have their chain featured. Despite these omissions, I have created a thorough list that provides any low-carb dieter with extensive options both in price and cuisine, helping you to meet your constantly evolving low-carb needs.

Yes, changes in America's eating habits are occurring at lightning speeds. Low-carb is the hot new consumer marketing niche. Likewise, most restaurants are going to make a fanfare of new low-carb menu items. I've included URLs for restaurant Web sites in this book so you can always go online and check the latest low-carb offerings any given chain might be featuring.

With this guide, you will finally be able to take your low-carb diet on the road, adhering to your carb restrictions whether you are two thousand miles from home or just stepping out for the evening. Get ready to put your social life into your diet because finally it is possible to lose weight and dine out.

Tips for Eating Out Low-Carb Style

As complicated as it may sound, eating low-carb is really very simple. You don't have to read many of the restaurants entries in this book to recognize a pattern. As long as you follow these basic low-carb rules, you'll be able to go anywhere.

1. **When estimating carb counts in an unfamiliar restaurant, you can use the general rule of thumb that all plain grilled, fried, boiled or broiled meats, seafood, eggs, cheeses, oils, and fats have zero carbs.** For the most part, a small green salad without croutons will have between four and six carb grams. An entrée-size lettuce salad (such as a Caesar) will have between six and ten grams. You should factor in between four and eight grams for most steamed legal vegetable side dishes. Where it gets tricky is estimating dressing and sauces. Stay away from anything that seems like it has added sugar or fruit juice. Many sauces and all gravies have some sort of thickening agents like cornstarch and flour. As long as there are no sweet agents in the sauce, the overall ration of thickener to sauce ingredients is usually small enough to be insubstantial—about two to four grams. Likewise, many cream sauces such as béarnaise or *beurre blanc* will qualify for low-carb status, but to be cautious, limit your intake unless you know exactly what went into preparing them.

2. **Choose vegetable side dishes according to the lowest carbs.** Green is better when it comes to low-carb vegetables. Order things like asparagus, broccoli, spinach, green beans, and leafy greens. Next best are veggies like

cauliflower, summer squash, tomatoes, bell peppers, mushrooms, and onions. Last on the veggie hierarchy are sweeter veggies like corn or carrots, although even with their higher carb count, they are healthy, fiber-filled carbs that have a much lower glycemic index than refined carbohydrates or starchy vegetables like potatoes or white rice.

3. **Avoid all starches—this means breads, potatoes, sweet potatoes, and rice.** Ask for double portions of steamed vegetables or green salad instead.

4. **Avoid all desserts unless they are sugar-free.** Even then, exercise caution. For instance, even if the filling of a sugar-free pie has minimal carbs, the crust still has a lot. Low-carb desserts at restaurants are few and far between, although Ruby Tuesday's and Houlihan's do currently have one dessert each on their menus.

5. **Beware of sweet sauces and glazes.** Something as innocent as grilled chicken can turn into a high-carb disaster if it's bathed in a sticky sweet fruit glaze or barbecue sauce.

6. **Be careful about small, high-carb additions to foods.** Did you know that the croutons on the average Caesar salad contain about ten grams of carbohydrates? When you're only allowed thirty or so carbs for the day, do you really want to spend a third on croutons? Look at your daily carb count range as a budget. You need to plan for the important things and not waste carbs on items that are not important to you.

7. **Order drinks carefully.** While many alcohols like vodka, rum, gin, bourbon, scotch, and whiskey have zero carbs, any of the sweeter liquors carry substantial carb counts. Be careful with mixers, too. No fruit juice,

tonic, sweet and sour mix, or regular sodas. Stick to diet soda or club soda. A squeeze of lemon or lime is okay.

8. **Sit as far from the bread basket as possible.** Bread is the nemesis of low-carb dieters. Ask your server to leave this dietary saboteur in the kitchen, or if you're dining with omnivorous friends, place it in front of them.

9. **Give yourself something to do while others indulge in dessert.** Try ordering an espresso or cappuccino or a nice cup of herb tea, with sugar-free sweeteners, of course.

10. **Carry plastic forks and knives in your car, purse, or briefcase.** No matter where you go, you can always get some sort of low-carb filled sandwich or burger that you can eat by tossing the bun. Having utensils makes the eating process immensely easier and neater. Even lettuce-wrapped foods are easier to eat with utensils than with your hands.

11. **Keep individual packets of low- or no-carb salad dressings with you.** In case the restaurant you're in lacks good dressing choices, you'll have your favorites with you.

12. **Don't let yourself get hungry. It will only cause you to overeat or go off your diet by the time you get to the restaurant.** Carry snacks like small bags of nuts, cheese, or low-carb energy bars with you for emergencies.

13. **If you must have the taste of a forbidden sauce or dressing, dip the tines of a fork in the sauce or dressing, then use the fork to pick up the food.** You'll get the essence of the taste you crave without all the accompanying carbs.

14. **Plan in advance which restaurant you'll be dining at and what food you will order.** If you already know what you want when you arrive at the restaurant, you won't be tempted to cheat. You won't even need to look at the menu.

Carbs: A Quick Reference Guide

GOOD CARBS VERSUS BAD CARBS

While the focus of this book is national and regional chain restaurants, don't forget that the best restaurants aren't chains or franchises. The best restaurants are the eateries—either small and casual or grand scale and deluxe—owned and operated by individuals and families who have a passion for food.

More than giving you specific menu recommendations for exactly what to order at any given restaurant, I hope this book will teach you how to eat out at any restaurant, confident that you won't sabotage your weight loss or maintenance goals.

For this reason, it's important to get familiar with the concept of the glycemic index in foods. Notice I didn't say you have to become a nutritionist. We're going to keep this simple and easy—you only need to be aware of the principle and how to choose foods accordingly. This way, if you ever find yourself in a restaurant situation where you have to eat some high-carb foods, you can minimize the damage to your weight loss goals.

While you'll find detailed information about the importance of a food's glycemic index in most of today's popular low-carb diet books, the simple explanation is the glycemic index of a food refers to how quickly after eating that food your body's insulin levels will spike and how high they will rise. Foods lower on the glycemic index digest more slowly than foods with high glycemic index numbers. Foods that digest slowly release sugar into your bloodstream at a slower rate, thereby reducing the body's need to produce as much insulin to help in metabolizing the food. Less insulin released usually translates to quicker weight loss.

> The Glycemic Index refers to the rate that different carbohydrates are transformed into sugars, released into the bloodstream, and absorbed by the body.

Some people are more sensitive to insulin than others; that's why one person can cheat frequently on a low-carb plan and still lose weight while others have to follow their plans to the letter. Don't worry, you don't have to memorize the glycemic index number for every food. Just remember this simple rule: natural foods tend to have lower glycemic indexes. Avoid processed foods whenever possible. Stick to real foods like meat, vegetables, fruits, dairy products, natural oils and butter, and whole grains. If you're going to eat bread, make it whole-grain, which digests slowly in your system, instead of white bread, which will spike your insulin levels like a rocket heading for the moon. Avoid anything with white sugar, which will do the same.

But this general rule isn't foolproof. Some natural foods also cause your insulin levels to spike. Avoid sweeteners like honey, maple syrup, molasses, and especially brown or white sugar. Pure starches must be avoided, too. A baked potato has a higher glycemic index than ice cream! Pass on potatoes, but if you are going to eat them, small, waxy red or yellow potatoes have a lower glycemic index than the fluffy, floury bakers served at most restaurants. The same goes for rice—opt for brown or wild rice and skip the sticky, starchy varieties served at most Asian restaurants.

Net Carbs Versus Total Carbs

As the editor of a low-carb Internet e-zine (get your free subscription at www.fabulousfoods.com), I frequently get e-mail from confused readers about net carb counts. "What is this mysterious net carb number, and do I need to count all the carbs in a dish or only the net carbs?" This is one of the most frequently asked questions by people trying to live the low-carb lifestyle.

Net carbs are fiber- and sugar alcohol–related carbohydrates that have a low glycemic index number. As use of the glycemic index has become more commonplace, low-carb dieters have started to calculate net carbs, as opposed to simply adding all carbs together as bad carbs. This is good news for low-carbers because it provides an extra handful or more of allowable carbs for their daily allotment. To determine a food's effective carb count, subtract the number of grams of fiber and/or sugar alcohols in the food from the total grams of carbohydrates. For example, a cup of steamed broccoli has a total carb count of 11.20 grams and a fiber count of 5.1 grams. Subtract 5.1 from 11.20, and you get 6.1 net grams of carbohydrates. Now doesn't 6.1 sound better than 11.20?

"But that sounds too good to be true," my readers lament.

In reality, it's not. The body does not process sugar alcohols (such as maltitol, which is used in making many low-carb candies) the way it does other carbs. Also, fiber in a food slows the digestion process, giving the food a lower rating on the glycemic index. The more complex the carbohydrate, the more natural fiber that remains in a food and the better it is for your low-carb diet. The more refined and processed a food is, the more it will make insulin levels rise.

How to Use This Book

I designed this book to be easy to use, whether you are at the restaurant and trying to decide what to order, or if you're planning in advance where to dine. Nobody wants to be the one person in a group who makes it difficult to choose a place to eat. With this guide, you will see that with very few exceptions, you can always find lots of great low-carb foods to eat, wherever you go.

RESTAURANT LISTINGS

The restaurants are divided into four categories:

FAST FOOD covers quick service restaurants (the kind where you order at a counter and get your food in a paper sack); for example, McDonald's, Taco Bell, and KFC.

CASUAL RESTAURANTS are usually inexpensive, often coffee-shop type—establishments like Denny's, IHOP, and Fuddrucker's.

MIDRANGE RESTAURANTS take food quality and ambiance up a notch, and most serve alcohol; Think eateries like TGI Friday's, Ruby Tuesday, or Steak and Ale.

UPSCALE RESTAURANTS represent the best that chain restaurants have to offer, with gourmet food made from fresh ingredients augmented by impressive wine lists.

RESTAURANT REVIEWS

Each restaurant review is divided into four parts:

THE GOOD presents the restaurant's merits, from a low-carb dining perspective.

THE BAD gives you the low-down on the menu obstacles and challenges that this restaurant presents to low-carb dieters.

THE UGLY refers to the menu items that can really put the brakes on your diet's success. Avoid them at all costs.

THE BEST THINGS TO EAT gives you specific low-carb menu recommendations.

Counting Carbs

Whenever possible, I have given the net carb count. Sometimes, as in the case of meats and cheeses, the net and total carb counts are the same.

Unless otherwise noted, the carb counts for salads do not include dressing. Don't panic! Unlike low-fat plans, most salad dressings are allowed on low-carb plans. Vinegar and oil are lowest in carbs of all. Blue cheese is also a dressing of choice. Depending on the exact recipe, it often contains zero carbs, but never has a substantial number. Ranch is usually a good bet, too, at zero to three grams per serving, depending on the brand. Most vinaigrettes are also low-carb, but beware and ask questions—some use fruit juice or other sweeter ingredients. For the most part, Asian-style salad dressings have more sugar than their western counterparts, and low-fat versions of salad dressing generally have higher carb counts and more sugar than their full-fat counterparts.

The carb counts in this book have been estimated to the nearest gram and to the best of my ability. Some restaurants have prepared detailed nutritional data on their menus and whenever possible I have given these figures; otherwise, I give approximate carb count ranges using the United States government's USDA Food Nutrient Database. As restaurants are somewhat secretive about giving out their proprietary recipes, it's impossible to be precise.

LOW-CARB EATING

How rigidly you follow the recommendations in this book depends on whether you are following the weight loss or maintenance phase of your diet. If you are trying to maintain rather than lose, you are can add additional

> **Note:** It is important for you to remember that the information in this book about restaurants and low-carb menus is subject to change and may vary from location to location. Consult the restaurant's Web site for the most current and up-to-the-minute information about menu changes, new low-carb promotions, and limited time specials.

carbs into your diet. Just remember to eat low on the glycemic index scale. Unless otherwise noted, my recommendations are suitable for the weight loss phases of most low-carb plans.

Look not only at the Good sections in each restaurant entrys but also the Bad and the Ugly. This way, you'll come to see how effectively these seemingly innocent little indiscretions undermine your diet and weight loss/maintenance goals. The information is meant to make you truly think and make a conscious decision about whether eating your burger on a bun as opposed to wrapped in lettuce is really worth it.

Use and reject the recommendations in this book accordingly. Different low-carb plans allow and restrict different foods. I have tried to accommodate as many as possible. That said, I assume you know which eating plan you are following—you know which foods your plan does and does not allow.

Even when the facts and figure are accurate, you must always acknowledge that certain variations are possible. Use carb counts as guideposts to keeping your diet on track, but don't live and die by knowing the precise number of carbs you consume, unless you have a medical condition that requires you to do so. Eat on the low end of your daily carb budget, and you'll be fine. M. Evans also publishes *Dr. Atkins's New Carbohydrate Gram Counter*.

This pocket-sized book is small enough to carry with you wherever you go, in case you ever really need to know the real facts

RATINGS AND SYMBOLS

Each review has icons that represent the general price range of items on their menu. This number usually refers to the average price of a protein entrée, as this is what most low-carbers will be ordering:

$	Under $5
$$	$5 to 10
$$$	$10 to $15
$$$$	$15 to $20
$$$$$	$20 and higher

Each restaurant is also rated by stars. The scope of this book is only interested in the number of quality low-carb choices a restaurant offers its customers. Restaurants are rated for their appropriateness for low-carbers, not on the taste, quality, or value of the food or service at the restaurant:

★	Hope you're not too hungry.
★★	A few solid choices.
★★★	No problem eating here.
★★★★	I can't believe how many menu choices I have!
★★★★★	Wow! You call this dieting?

A wine glass denotes that beer, wine, and/or alcohol is served at all the locations in a given chain.

A half wine glass lets you know that only some of the restaurants in that chain serve alcohol.

Fast Food Restaurants

ARBY'S
★★★ | $
www.arbys.com
Found throughout the United States, parts of Canada, and in limited international locations (Qatar, United Arab Emirates, Mexico, Turkey, and Egypt).
Claim to Fame: roast beef sandwiches

THE GOOD
Arby's serves a variety of low-carb salads. It's new Arby's Low Carbys menu gives you the best of Arby's sandwiches, without the bread.

THE BAD
Leaving the bread or roll on your sandwich will pack an extra twenty-two to thirty carb grams onto your daily count. Save an extra four to five carbs by leaving the croutons off salads. Even the low-carb tortilla-wrapped Arby's Low Carbys sandwiches have at least seventeen grams of net carbs. Better to order the breadless versions. Chicken at Arby's is coated and fried, so even the breadless chicken sandwiches contain sixteen carb grams.

THE UGLY
Don't even think about ordering fries, onion rings, breaded jalapenos, mozzarella sticks, or, especially, baked potatoes. Ditto desserts and Arby's sweet shakes. Stick to salads and protein, and you'll stick to your low-carb eating plan.

The Best Things to Eat at Arby's: The Caesar side salad contains only four carbs; double that number for a meal-sized Caesar or chicken Caesar salad. You only have to account for nine grams when enjoying a turkey club salad. Top your salad with a serving of light mayonnaise or Caesar dressing for only one carb. Blue cheese, buttermilk ranch, reduced-calorie Italian dressing, and Arby's Horsey Sauce contain three carbs per serving each.

The Low Carbys menu also offers a wide variety of breadless roast beef, ham, and turkey sandwiches, all under six grams of carbs. Most have only one or two grams (except for the chicken, see above).

Breakfast: Any of Arby's breakfast sandwiches are low-carb if you eliminate the bread. Order yours with extra egg for a more substantial morning meal. Keep in mind, however, that "eggs" at Arby's (like many fast food restaurants) are preformed patties that also contain milk solids and two carb grams per "egg."

A&W
★★ | $

www.awrestaurants.com

Over 800 restaurants found throughout the Unites States.

Claim to Fame: root beer, burgers

THE GOOD
The terrific diet root beer here is a real treat for zero carbs.

THE BAD
Everything else on the menu is high-carb, except for bunless sandwiches and burgers. There are no legal side dishes—just fries, chili fries, cheese fries, and onion rings.

THE UGLY
A&W offers some seriously high-carb ice cream treats that low-carbers can't have.

The Best Things to Eat at A&W: Stick to breadless burgers or grilled chicken sandwiches topped with favorite no- and low-carb toppings like bacon, cheese, tomatoes, and onions. Hot dog fans can order bunless dogs, with or without cheese and/or chili. Get a dog with both for about six to eight net carbs. Of course, if you don't bring along a fork and knife, it will be messy to eat.

BAJA FRESH
★★ | $
www.bajafresh.com
Over 300 restaurants in twenty-six states, with concentrations on east and west coasts.
Claim to Fame: healthy, fresh baja-style Mexican food

THE GOOD
"Customers have always been able to customize our menu to make it compatible with whatever diet they follow," says Greg Dollarhyde, President/CEO of Baja Fresh. Since the menu items at this popular chain are based around fresh, healthy grilled meat, you can always find something to eat with some simple substitutions and omissions.

THE BAD
Baja Fresh's new steak and chicken picado were developed for the "one in seven Americans following a high protein diet." While these menu items may be high in protein, they are also high in carbs. A press release on the dishes proudly proclaims they have less than thirty-two grams of carbs! While this is less than traditional Mexican fare, it will still break the bank of most low-carb plans, although to be fair, these are mostly healthy carbs from veggies.

THE UGLY
Avoid anything with tortillas, tortilla chips, and/or rice. Beans will add carbs to your daily count, but many low-carb plans allow healthy, fiber-rich beans.

The Best Things to Eat at Baja Fresh: Your best bet is the Side-by-Side meal consisting of charbroiled chicken and a side salad, served with guacamole, pico de gallo, jack cheese, avocado slices, and fat-free salsa verde dressing, for sixteen total carb grams. Next best is the Baja Ensalada—

romaine lettuce, charbroiled chicken, tortilla strips, and pico de gallo, all tossed to order and topped with shaved cheese and tomato slices, for seventeen grams. Leaving off the tortilla strips makes this the best menu item of all to order—about nine net carbs (salad dressing and salsa not counted in carb count). You can also custom-order your own food. Choose grilled steak, chicken, or fish served on a bed of lettuce. Add some cheese, sour cream, and fresh salsas, and you've got a great low-carb, baja-style meal.

BLIMPIE
★★★ | $
www.blimpie.com
About 1,600 restaurants across the United States and in thirteen countries.
Claim to Fame: submarine sandwiches and salads

THE GOOD
It's ironic that Blimpie's, a restaurant whose reputation was made by serving great submarine sandwiches, was one of the first national chains to jump on the low-carb bandwagon. Blimpie president and CEO Jeff Endervelt, who lost weight on a low-carb plan himself, says the chain plans to continue to update and add options to the BCC (Blimpie Carb Counter) menu regularly. Atkins Nutritionals, SoBe Beverages, and French's mustard all cooperated in the creation of the new menu that includes tasty condiments, low-carb breads, brownies, chips, and gourmet sugar-free beverages. In addition to Blimpie's Low-Carb menu, you can remove the bread from most other Blimpie sandwiches and stay within most low-carb diet guidelines.

THE BAD
The breads on most sandwiches will break the carb count bank, so you're better off ordering salads, with the exception of the sandwiches on Blimpie's innovative new Carb Counter menu.

THE UGLY
Stay away from the fresh-baked cookies (although Blimpie's does offer a low-carb brownie). Side dishes like potato salads and macaroni salad are also off limits. Even the cole slaw has thirteen carbs per serving.

The Best Things to Eat at Blimpie's: Anything from the Carb-Counter Menu will fit into most diets. Try the buffalo chicken salad for five net carbs per serving or the antipasto salad for seven grams. You can choose from a number of low-carb sandwiches. The following carb counts are for six-inch sandwiches: seven grams net carbs for turkey, provolone, and French's GourMayo chipotle; the roast beef, cheddar, and French's GourMayo wasabi, or the buffalo chicken, provolone, and French's GourMayo sun-dried tomato low-carb sandwiches each run eight net carbs; for 8.5 grams net carbs order the ham, swiss, and French's mustard. Pair your low-carb sandwich with Atkins Crunchers Chips for about three grams of net carbs per serving. Budget carefully and you can even indulge your sweet tooth with a Blimpie Carb Counter Brownie at about five net carbs per serving. Wash it all down with SoBe Lean drinks that contain only one net carb gram per eight ounce serving and no aspartame.

Best Dressings/Condiments: Blimpie offers a number of tasty choices when it comes to salad dressings and sandwich fixings. The oil and vinegar topping for a six-inch sub contains only a half-gram of carbs. Pesto has only one carb and the Caesar and cracked peppercorn dressings weigh in at two carbs per serving. Even if you splurge on guacamole, it will only cost your daily carb budget seven carb grams.

> **TIP:** Blimpie wants to help you stay on your low-carb diet—even when you eat elsewhere. Their Web site offers low-carbers a free downloadable daily carb-counting journal you can print from your own computer. Use this freebie to track your daily intake. Writing down everything you eat can be a powerful motivator in curbing indulgences. The journal pages have plenty of space to list foods consumed for breakfasts, lunches, dinners, and snacks, along with the net effective carb counts for those foods. You can also keep track of which vitamins and supplements you take, the amount and types of exercise you do, and other notes you might find useful to refer to later on.

BOSTON MARKET
★★★ | $–$$
www.bostonmarket.com
Over 600 restaurants in 28 states, with concentrations on the East Coast, Florida, midwest, southwest, and California.

Claim to Fame: rotisserie chicken

THE GOOD
Boston Market makes good, old-fashioned comfort food, just like you might make at home if you had the time or inclination. You'll get roasted meats, fresh vegetables, salads, and soups; in other words, value-priced traditional American fare. Order a quarter- or half-chicken meal, rotisserie turkey, or even Boston hearth ham, paired with two or three legal side dishes for a custom-made, low-carb meal, just the way you like it. You can also buy Boston Market whole rotisserie chickens, and hand-carved turkey and ham in family sizes to keep in your fridge for quick low-carb lunches and snacks.

THE BAD
A 5.5-ounce serving of meatloaf at sixteen carbs isn't the biggest dietary sin, but there are so many other good things to eat at Boston Market, why waste carbs on ordinary meatloaf? The oriental grilled chicken salad will set you back fifty-eight carb grams. Order yours without noodles and you can shave thirty-eight carb grams from that total. The chicken tortilla salad at forty-six grams isn't harmless, either. Order it without chips or dressing and the carb count lowers to twenty-two grams.

THE UGLY
Stay away from the cole slaw—at thirty carb grams per 6.5 ounce serving, there's just way too much sugar. Of course, avoid all potatoes, pastas, sandwiches (unless you're prepared to toss the bread), and desserts (with

the possible exception of the fruit salad, depending on
your individual diet plan).

The Best Things to Eat at Boston Market: The roast
chicken rules. For only four grams of carbohydrates, you
can eat half a roast chicken with the skin on! For chicken
with the lowest carb grams, order a quarter roast dark
meat chicken without the skin, or a serving of marinated
grilled chicken for only a single carb gram. A five-ounce
serving of roast turkey breast contains just three carbs. You
can add an order of chicken gravy to any dish for just two
additional carbs. Boston Market's chunky chicken salad is
also a good bargain at four grams per six-ounce serving.
An order of honey-glazed ham will cost your carb budget
ten grams—not a terrible price to pay if you crave this
choice.

Low-carb sides of note at Boston Market include green
beans at four carbs, the steamed vegetable medley at six
grams, the green bean casserole nine grams, and creamed
spinach at eleven grams. If you leave the toppings off
a serving of chicken or turkey tortilla soup, you'll only
consume seven carb grams. A serving of chicken noodle
soup has only eight carbs. Pick out the noodles and the
carb count lowers. The side and entrée sizes of the Boston
Market's Caesar salad contain thirteen and seventeen
grams of carbs respectively, but pick out the croutons and
you'll save about nine grams. If your plan allows fruit, a
six-ounce serving of Boston Market's fruit salad has only
sixteen carb grams.

BURGER KING
★★★ | $

www.burgerking.com

Found in the United States and fifty-eight countries.

Claim to Fame: charbroiled burgers prepared "your way"

THE GOOD

Burger King offers several direct off-the-menu items that fit nicely into low-carb plans, and all of Burger King's sandwiches, are now available served on a bed of lettuce. The fire-grilling cooking techniques used by this mega-chain give the fare a great flavor, especially for inexpensive fast food.

THE BAD

Get careless and leave the buns on the burgers and chicken sandwiches, and you'll raise your daily carb count by a whopping forty-five carb grams each. Eating the sourdough bread in breakfast sandwiches will cost you twenty-eight grams and the bread portion of the breakfast Croissandwich will set you back twenty-two carbs. Eat the fillings, not the breads. Avoid the chicken tenders—a five-piece serving packs thirteen grams of carbs and an eight-piece serving weighs in at twenty grams. Because of its breading, Burger King's original chicken sandwich contains thirteen grams of carbohydrates. Stay away from the fish sandwich, too; even without the bun, you'll still consume sixteen grams of carbs. A bunless BK Veggie sandwich with full-fat mayonnaise will cost you eighteen grams of carbs (nineteen grams with fat-free mayo).

THE UGLY

If the temptation of some of the best fast-food French fries in the world is too much for you to resist, don't go to Burger King. A small order of fries will cost your carb budget 29 grams. Forget desserts, too.

The Best Things to Eat at Burger King: For ordering straight off the menu, the chicken caesar salad (minus croutons and dressing) at only five carb grams is the best bet. Add Caesar salad dressing for only two grams of carbs. Skip the croutons, and you'll save fourteen grams of insulin-raising carbs. A Burger King side salad has only five grams of dietary carbs. Your best dressing bet is Kraft's ranch dressing at one carb per one-ounce. serving. Be sure to order the full-fat version of the ranch dressing; the fat-free contains more sugars and therefore more carbs—a hefty nine grams per single ounce portion. One-ounce servings of the light Italian or the creamy Caesar salad dressings will only cost you two carb grams.

Burger King is now offering low-carb, lettuce-wrapped versions of their most popular sandwiches, including the Original Whopper, Chicken Whopper, Bacon Whopper, Double Whopper, Whopper Jr., and the new fire-Grilled Angus Steak Burger; all can be ordered with or without cheese without affecting carbs counts. The low-carb style "sandwiches" at Burger King contain less than five carb grams each, providing that you order them without ketchup or mayo.

Burger King also offers some interesting chicken sandwiches that will fit into most low-carb plans, providing you toss the bread. A grilled chicken Caesar club or the Santa Fe chicken baguette has only six grams of carbs, a savory mustard chicken baguette has seven, and a BBQ Chicken Baguette has eight grams.

Breakfast: Burger King's breakfast sandwiches, *sans* bread, of course, make good low-carb ways to start the day. Toss the bread and you can eat a sourdough bacon, ham, or sausage, egg and cheese sandwich with only two carb grams and a ham, egg, and cheese Croissandwich at three grams.

CAPTAIN D'S
★★★ | $–$$
www.captainds.com
Over 550 restaurants in 22 states in the southern half of
the United States.
Claim to Fame: seafood/fish and chips

THE GOOD:
The Captain's Broiler menu gives low-carbers lots of
choices of healthy broiled seafood—low-carb, low fat,
and delicious. You'll also find a few good side dish
choices here.

THE BAD
Avoid hushpuppies and, as always, the potatoes—both
baked and fried. The cheese sticks and jalapeno bites
contain breading that brings their carb counts to an
unacceptable level. Ditto the cole slaw—like most com-
mercially made versions, it has too much sugar.

THE UGLY
The desserts can do you in, so don't even think about
the Captain's pies or cheesecakes.

The Best Things to Eat at Captain D's: Pick anything
on the Captain's Broiler menu that includes fish, shrimp,
chicken, or combinations thereof. The meat portion of
the meal contains little or no carbs. Other great low-carb
choices include Pacific Northwest salmon or broiled New
Zealand orange roughy (zero carbs). For side dishes choose
the tossed salad (about five net carbs) with a low-carb
dressing like blue cheese or ranch, or an order of green
beans (about four net carbs).

CARL'S JR.
★★★ | $
www.carlsjr.com
Over 1,000 restaurants in the western United States.
Claim to Fame: burgers

THE GOOD
Carl's Jr. recognizes the importance of the low-carb market, as evidenced by their new lettuce-wrapped Six Dollar Low-Carb Burger, which in reality costs a whole lot less than six bucks. Carl's also offers some decent low-carb salads and lots of sandwich options if you have the willpower to toss the bread. No willpower? No problem. Just ask for any of Carl's Jr. sandwiches "low-carb style" and your food will come wrapped in lettuce instead of on a bun. Carl's (along with sister restaurants Hardee's) saw such success with their low-carb style burgers they quickly added a low-carb breakfast to their menus.

THE BAD
Read the menu carefully. Even with eliminating the bun, many Carl's Jr. sandwiches have high-carb counts because of breading. Some chicken sandwiches are grilled, others breaded and fried (avoid the latter). Any of the "crispy" chicken sandwiches are breaded. Even without the bun, a Carl's crispy ranch chicken sandwich packs twenty-nine grams of carbs. Also, beware of Carl's "Western" sandwiches. They come topped with ten carb grams worth of breaded onion rings. A bunless breaded Fish Sandwich will still set you back twenty-four grams of carbs.

THE UGLY
As usual, avoid all breads, desserts, and potatoes—both fried and baked.

The Best Things to Eat at Carl's Jr.: The Six-Dollar Low-Carb Burger at just six grams of carbs makes a satisfying entrée. The charbroiled chicken salad to go has eighteen grams of (mostly) healthy carbs—in other words, carbs from veggies. In the breadless sandwich category, your best bets are the Famous Star Hamburger at seven carb grams or the Famous Bacon Cheeseburger, mushroom Swiss burger, or Six-Dollar Bacon Cheeseburger at eight grams each. Best of all is the charbroiled sirloin steak sandwich; if you don't eat the bun and leave off the onion rings, it has only four grams of carbs. Chicken lovers should choose the charbroiled chicken club sandwich at eight carbs without the bread, and the charbroiled Santa Fe chicken sandwich at ten grams.

Breakfast: Breakfast at Carl's is easy, just order the Low-Carb Breakfast Bowl. For just six total grams of carbohydrates, you get a bowl filled with legal breakfast favorites: two folded eggs, a sausage patty, a slice of Swiss cheese, and a "loaded omelet" made with sausage, crumbled bacon, shredded cheddar cheese, and topped with more crumbled bacon and shredded cheese. If that sounds like too much breakfast for you, you can also order eggs and breakfast meats à la carte, meaning there is no temptation to eat the bread. An order of scrambled eggs has just one carb gram and sausage patties run two carbs per patty.

CHICK-FIL-A
★★★ | $
www.chickfila.com
Thousands of stores in thirty-seven states, mostly in shopping malls.
Claim to Fame: chicken sandwiches

THE GOOD
Chick-fil-A is committed to honoring their customers' special requests. As such, you can ask for any of their sandwiches wrapped in lettuce instead of on a bun. Another plus to eating here is that all Chick-fil-A salads are "modular"—the ingredients are grouped together so it's easy to pick off the foods you don't want.

THE BAD
A 3.7-ounce portion of the regular breaded Chick-fil-A has ten grams of carbs. Order your chicken charbroiled and you'll save nine grams. Avoid the Chick-N-Strips and Nuggets at fourteen and twelve carb grams per serving respectively. You'll also want to steer clear of the carrot raisin salad (twenty-two carb grams) and the cole slaw (fourteen grams). Even the chicken soup is a no-no. A large portion contains thirty-seven grams of carbs. Leave the tortilla strips off your salad and you'll save nine carbs.

THE UGLY
Even the small waffle potato fries pack thirty-seven grams of carbs. Beware of some salad dressings, too: the reduced-fat raspberry vinaigrette dressing packs a whopping fifteen grams of carbs per serving, fourteen for the fat-free honey dijon. The thousand island contains just five grams of carbs, but there are better choices. Desserts are strictly off limits, as they'll cost you anywhere between twenty-eight and fifty-one grams of carbs.

The Best Things to Eat at Chick-fil-A: A charbroiled chicken filet has only one carb gram. Pair it with a side salad, and your entire meal will only contain two grams of carbohydrates. The charbroiled chicken salad, at only nine carbs, is another terrific entrée. The tasty charbroiled Southwest chicken salad weighs in with seventeen grams of carbs, but you can shave this number down to eight by foregoing the tortilla strips. Top any of your salads with honey-roasted sunflower seeds for just three additional grams of healthy carbs. Choose salad dressings wisely (see above). Your best bets are Caesar, buttermilk ranch, or blue cheese, at just one gram per serving or lite Italian and spicy dressings for just two grams.

Breakfast: A plain biscuit at Chick-fil-A contains thirty-eight carb grams. Toss the bread and you can order the bacon, egg, and cheese biscuit—or any combination thereof—and not consume any carbs! The same breakfast with sausage instead of bacon will run you five grams of carbs.

CHURCH'S CHICKEN
★ | $
www.churchs.com
Over 1,500 restaurants in twenty-eight states, Puerto Rico, and nine other countries.
Claim to Fame: fried chicken

THE GOOD
The fried chicken at Church's, especially if you have the willpower to remove the batter and skin, is remarkably low in carbohydrates. Even if you cheat and leave batter and skin on, Church's chicken has a relatively low-carb count, so a piece or two won't completely blow things. A regular serving of cole slaw has an effective carb count of only eight grams, making it a decent side order choice. This count is significantly lower than most other restaurants' cole slaws. Kudos to Church's for keeping unnecessary carbs and sugar out of our diet.

THE BAD
The carb counts on the majority of side dishes are too high for most low-carb dieters—even dishes that seem like they should be reasonable choices. For instance, a regular-sized serving of okra at Church's contains nineteen carb grams, a single ear of corn on the cob has twenty-four grams. Beware of some of Church's sauces, too. A single-serving package of Purple Pepper Sauce contains twelve grams of carbs, with Sweet and Sour sauce following close behind at eight grams, followed in short order by BBQ sauce at seven grams and honey mustard sauce at four.

THE UGLY
While the traditional fried chicken at Church's won't break the daily carb budget, an order of Tender Crunchers at thirty-two carbs or Krispy Tender Strips

will. Never order the chicken fried steak, as this dish packs a whopping thirty-six grams of carbs. Snacks will cost you, too—four jalapeno Cheese Bombers will set you back twenty-nine carb grams and a regular-sized order of Sweet Corn Nuggets packs in some thirty carb grams.

Of course, forget potatoes and bread; a regular-sized order of French fries will set you back twenty-nine grams of carbs, mashed potatoes have fourteen grams, and a single honey butter biscuit has twenty-six grams. Desserts are strictly off limits, too. A serving of strawberry cream cheese pie has thirty-two grams of carbs, a piece of double lemon pie has thirty-nine grams, and a slice of apple pie has forty-one grams.

The Best Things to Eat at Church's: The best bet at Church's is the fried chicken with the batter and skin removed. A chicken breast consumed this way has just one carb gram, a leg 1.25, a wing two, and a thigh three grams. Even if you don't have the willpower to remove the batter and skin, the carb counts remain relatively low: four grams for a breast, two for a leg, five for a thigh, and eight for a wing. While this last number may sound surprising, it isn't when you consider the wing's surface area to meat ratio. Unfortunately, as of this writing, Church's doesn't offer salads (except cole slaw), so an order of collard greens at five grams is a viable and healthy alternative. At only one carb gram per packet, Church's creamy jalapeno sauce makes a good way to spice up your meal.

DEL TACO
★ | $
www.deltaco.com
Currently in thirteen states, with concentrations on the western United States.
Claim to Fame: Mexican fast food

THE GOOD
You'll be able to piece together something to eat at Del Taco, with some substitutions and menu item omissions, although low-carbers are hardly this restaurant's core market. According to a Del Taco spokesperson, Del Taco customers like Del Taco food the way it is, so why change a good thing?

THE BAD
All menu items are off limits for low-carb dieters; however, you can leave out a few ingredients and make it work.

THE UGLY
Most everything on this menu is high-carb. Read item descriptions carefully and eliminate bread, tortillas, and rice, and you'll do fine at Del Taco.

The Best Things to Eat at Del Taco: The regular taco salad at ten grams of carbs is your best bet at this restaurant, which offers limited low-carb choices at best. The Macho Beef or Del Classic chicken burritos contain only grilled meats and low-carb veggies like lettuce, tomatoes, and onions, and carbless condiments like cheese and sour cream; so as long as you don't eat the tortilla, they make good entrée choices. The burgers are good, too, minus the special sauce and without the buns.

DOMINO'S PIZZA
★ | $
www.dominos.com
Found throughout the United States and internationally.
Claim to Fame: pizza

THE GOOD
About the only thing Domino's has to offer low-carb dieters are its chicken wings, unless you have the willpower to eat only the pizza toppings and leave the crust. If you can do this, you're a stronger person than I am.

THE BAD
Pizza crusts will sabotage your diet in a heartbeat. If you can't resist, then resist a visit to Dominos.

THE UGLY
Most everything on this menu is high-carb, from the pizzas to the breadsticks.

The Best Things to Eat at Domino's: The buffalo chicken wings at a half carb gram per wing are the best bet, closely followed by the barbecue wings at 1.58 carb grams per wing.

EL POLLO LOCO
★★★ | $–$$
www.elpolloloco.com
Over 300 restaurants in four states: California, Arizona, Nevada, and Texas.
Claim to Fame: marinated grilled chicken

THE GOOD
With grilled chicken being the default menu item at El Pollo Loco, you can rest assured you'll always get something tasty, filling, and satisfying to eat. El Pollo Loco also serves low-carb salads, and you can dress up meals with lots of legal salsas and extras like sour cream and guacamole.

THE BAD
Forget dessert; a single churro has eighteen grams of carbs, less than I would have expected, but still a diet buster. If you must eat tortillas, the 4.5-inch corn tortilla contains eight carb grams, and a six-inch corn tortilla has fourteen grams. Forego the Spanish rice and save thirty-four carb grams. An order of pinto beans will cost your carb budget twenty-six grams and a mere 2.8 ounces of tortilla chips will set you back forty-eight carbs.

THE UGLY
A twelve-inch flour tortilla weighs in at fifty-one grams of carbohydrates. The most carb-friendly burrito at El Pollo Loco, the Chicken Lover's Burrito, still has fifty-five carb grams. Be careful with sides—an order of French fries comes with sixty-one carb grams, thirty-five grams for smoky black beans, thirty for potato salad, twenty-five grams for macaroni and cheese, and twenty-one grams for mashed potatoes (add another fifteen grams for gravy). Even the cole slaw and corn cobbette are off limits for

most low-carbers, at twelve and eighteen carb grams respectively. Some El Pollo Loco's also offer menu items from Foster's Freeze franchise. If soft-serve ice cream and milkshakes are weaknesses, beware!

The Best Things to Eat at El Pollo Loco: The grilled chicken is undoubtedly the best thing to eat here. At zero carbs, you can chow down to your heart's content. Need variety? Add an order of fresh vegetables for only six grams, a garden salad for eight grams, or a Caesar salad with dressing for eighteen grams. With the exception of the Thousand Island (seven grams per 1.5 ounce serving), none of El Pollo Loco's salad dressings will cost your carb budget more than two grams. In fact, a half-ounce serving of the creamy cilantro dressing has zero carbs and the creamy chipotle only has one. Spice up your chicken and salads with low-carb extras like sour cream and any of El Pollo Loco's salsas and hot sauces for just one extra carb per serving. Add a one-ounce serving of guacamole for just three extra-healthy carbs.

FATBURGER
★★ | $$
www.fatburger.com
More than fifty restaurants in twenty states, with concentrations in the west, southwest, and east.

Claim to Fame: hamburgers

THE GOOD
While they've been serving bunless sandwiches for some time now, Fatburger is just starting to promote their low-carb offerings under the name "Fatkins." Director of marketing Elaine Patel comments, "Fatkins makes it easy for Fatburger fans who are counting their carbohydrates and don't want to feel guilty about enjoying their favorite hamburger. You might say we got rid of our buns so they don't have to worry about theirs."

THE BAD
Forget about fries, chili fries, or onion rings.

THE UGLY
Fatburger's real ice cream milkshakes may be delicious, but they have no place on a low-carb plan.

The Best Things to Eat at Fatburger: Order anything from the "Fatkins" menu—meaning bunless sandwiches. You'll get the same great taste and condiments as on Fatburger's regular burgers while curbing carbs. Top your regular 1/3-pound Fatkins-style burger with mustard, relish, onions, pickles, tomato, and mayonnaise for about five net carbs. For zero additional carbs, feel free to add cheese or even a fried egg to your burger. Those with smaller appetites can order a smaller "Baby Fat" burger. If beef isn't your thing you can also get Fatkins-style turkey burgers or grilled chicken.

GRANDY'S
★★★ | $–$$
www.grandys.com
Hundreds of restaurants in fourteen states, with concentrations in the midwest, south, and southwest.
Claim to Fame: fast food country cooking

THE GOOD
While low-carb offerings here are somewhat sparse, you will find a few viable options.

THE BAD
The menu is laden with breaded, fried things that will undermine low-carb diets: chicken-fried steak, chicken-fried chicken, and breaded catfish nuggets.

THE UGLY
Side dishes are starch city—mashed potatoes, French fries, and seasoned rice, not to mention corn on the cob and sweet, carb-filled baked beans.

The Best Things to Eat at Grandy's: Luckily, Grandy's serves a southwestern grilled chicken salad that fits nicely in a low-carb diet. Skip the croutons and go for a low-carb dressing like oil and vinegar, ranch, or blue cheese, and the effective carb counts should be in the ten-to-twelve gram range. You can also get a small green or garden salad (about four to six net carbs). In the entrée category, try the Southwestern grilled chicken (about two carbs) paired with an order of green beans (about four net carbs).

HARDEE'S
★★★ | $
www.hardees.com
Found in thirty-two U.S. (mostly in the south and east) and in eleven other countries.
Claim to Fame: burgers

THE GOOD
If you've ever been to Carl's Jr., the menu at Hardee's will seem uncannily familiar. The two restaurant chains are owned by the same corporation and likewise sport similar, although not identical, menu choices. CKE Restaurants are well aware of the impact low-carb dieters have on their bottom line and were one of the first chains to jump on the low-carb bandwagon. First came low-carb, lettuce-wrapped burgers, which proved so popular, Hardee's (and sister restaurants Carl's Jr.) quickly followed up with the fast food industry's first Low-Carb Breakfast Bowl.

THE BAD
Unlike their West Coast counterpart, Carl's Jr., Hardee's doesn't currently offer any salad options, which means there's really no side orders for low-carbers. Hopefully, they will rethink this and add more green options to their menu in the future.

THE UGLY
The worst carb offenders on the Hardee's menu are shakes. A large vanilla shake packs 123 grams of carbohydrates; make it a chocolate shake and you've got 171 carb grams. A Strawberry shake weighs in at 174 grams of insulin-spiking carbs. Of course, potatoes, breads, and desserts are strictly off limits.

The Best Things to Eat at Hardee's: The lettuce-wrapped 1/3-pound Low-Carb Thickburger, at five carb grams, is the default low-carb menu choice at Hardee's, but keep in mind that Hardee's staff will happily fix any of the restaurant's burgers or sandwiches "low-carb style." Ask for them lettuce-wrapped and Hardee's sandwiches provide good carb bargains: Big Roast Beef sandwich at 0.2 carb grams; the Big Hot Ham 'N' Cheese at 2.1; the mushroom Swiss burger at 4.2; the 1/3 lb. bacon cheeseburger at 6.1; the double bacon cheeseburger at 7.1; and the charbroiled chicken sandwich at 8.8.

Breakfast: The Hardee's Low-Carb Breakfast Bowl is a hearty mix of two folded eggs, a sausage patty, a slice of Swiss cheese, and a "loaded omelet" made with sausage, crumbled bacon, shredded cheddar cheese, and topped with more crumbled bacon and shredded cheese. Wow, that's a lot of food for only six total grams of carbs!

I'm not sure why you'd want to order anything but the low-carb breakfast at Hardee's, but if you want variety, simply throw out the biscuit or croissant and chow down on the fillings in the following breakfast items: the sausage egg and cheese or the loaded omelet biscuits contain just one carb each; the bacon, egg, and cheese and ham, egg, and cheese biscuits have two carbs; the Sunrise croissant with bacon or ham has two carbs or with sausage for three carbs; the Frisco breakfast sandwich's filling totals only two carbs. You can also order sides of breakfast meats: ham, bacon, or sausage for zero carbs; a chicken filet for one carb; or scrambled or folded eggs for one carb.

IN-N-OUT BURGER
★ | $
www.inandout.com
Over 140 restaurants in California, Nevada, and Arizona.
Claim to Fame: burgers

THE GOOD
While they're only found in limited states and only offer low-carbers one option—lettuce-wrapped burgers, the quality of these fast-food restaurants is so high they merit a mention. Be aware the "protein style" burgers are not on In-n-Out's very limited menu; you have to ask for them.

THE BAD
At fifty-four grams of carbohydrates per serving, the French fries are off limits to low-carbers, but your non-low-carbing dining companions will appreciate the fact that In-n-Out makes their fries fresh from real potatoes, not like the frozen, precut fries that dominate the fast food industry.

THE UGLY
Order water, unsweetened tea, coffee, or (if your diet allows it) a diet Coca-Cola to drink. While delicious, the vanilla, chocolate, or strawberry milkshakes at In-n-Out contain 78, 93, and 91 carb grams, respectively.

The Best Things to Eat at In-n-Out: Ask for any of In-N-Out's burgers to be served "protein style," and you'll get their same famous, quality burgers wrapped in lettuce instead of on a bun. Served this way, a single hamburger, cheeseburger, or Double Double (double meat, double cheese) has only eleven grams of carbs. Those with bigger appetites can order a three-by-three or even four-by-four protein-style burgers. The numbers refer to how many meat and cheese patties make up the burger.

JACK IN THE BOX
★★★ | $
www.jackinthebox.com
Currently in sixteen states throughout the west and parts of the midwest and south.
Claim to Fame: hamburgers, tacos, and Jack.

THE GOOD
Jack in the Box has introduced a new "Drive Through Dieting" promotion that allows you to order any burger or sandwich without the bun. Jack will serve up your meal in a resealable box along with a fork and knife, much neater than trying to manipulate a lettuce-wrapped burger in your hands. You'll also find some solid salad choices here.

THE BAD
The Southwest chicken salad starts at eighteen grams of carbs but if you eat the spicy corn sticks that come with it, you'll consume an additional twenty carbs. The creamy Southwest dressing will add another seven, making this an unwise salad choice. Even served bunless, Jack's spicy chicken sandwich contains fifteen carb grams, so does a regular sized taco— not the worst things you can eat, but Jack in the Box certainly offers better choices. The usual fast food diet culprits are also lurking here, with some creative new off-limit additions like batter-fried fish and chicken strips, egg rolls, onion rings, seasoned curly fries, and cheese-stuffed, batter-fried jalapenos.

THE UGLY
Beware of the Asian sesame salad dressing: 2¹/₂ ounces contains a surprising twenty grams of carbs. The items in the dessert and shakes category at Jack in the Box range from thirty-four carb grams in a slice of cheesecake to 199 grams in a strawberry

banana ice cream shake. In other words, they are all diet busters.

The Best Things to Eat at Jack in the Box: Most of Jack's burgers and sandwiches served low-carb style or bunless carry marginal carb counts: Jumbo Jack: two grams; Ultimate Cheeseburger: three grams; Bacon Ultimate Cheeseburger or Sourdough Jack Burger: four grams; bacon bacon cheeseburger or sourdough grilled chicken club: five grams. In the salad category, your best bet is the side salad at four grams. Jack's Ultimate Salads make good low-carb meals, but be careful with dressing choices and add-ons. The chicken club salad has only twelve grams of carbs, but add croutons and you've packed on another eleven grams, not to mention bacon ranch dressing at five and slivered almonds at four grams. The Asian chicken salad has only eighteen carbs, but add wonton strips and slivered almonds and you've added another seventeen carbs. Best to order your salad served with lite ranch dressing (three carbs) or traditional ranch dressing (four grams).

Breakfast: Don't expect an ultralow-carb or no-carb breakfast at Jack in the Box. A bunless version of Jack's Extreme Sausage Sandwich contains nine carb grams, an Ultimate Breakfast Sandwich (*sans* bread) weighs in at fourteen grams.

JODY MARONI'S SAUSAGE KINGDOM
★★★ | $
www.jodymaroni.com
Found in many airports, as well as West Coast locations.
Claim to Fame: gourmet sausage

THE GOOD

This is still a small chain, but growing—keep your eyes peeled for Jody Maroni's in airports, highway rest stops, and shopping malls. Jody Maroni's is very proud of the fact that you can order any of their delicious gourmet sausages wrapped in lettuce instead of a bun. Low-carb dieters are thrilled because Jody's sausages make a tasty alternative to lettuce-wrapped fast food burgers. They're all natural, use lean cuts of meat, and are nitrate- and MSG-free (monosodium glutamate). Depending on which diet you're following, Jody Maroni's roasted corn salad makes a nutritious and flavorful side dish. While we couldn't get exact nutritional data on this item, ordered without dressing, it won't do serious damage to your daily carb count as it consists of lettuce, tomatoes, peppers, onions, and just enough roasted corn kernels to give it an extraordinary flavor.

THE BAD

The only type of sausage that has any carbs to speak of is the smoked chicken Cubana with plaintains and rice (five carbs per sausage). The other varieties have between zero and three grams of carbs, if you don't eat the bun. At Jody Maroni's, you can even be bad and be good.

THE UGLY

You're at Jody Maroni's to eat sausage. Get it? With the exception of mustard and some grilled onions and peppers or sauerkraut, you pretty much have to avoid everything else. No fries, no chili, no nachos, roasted corn, churros, or pretzels.

The Best Things to Eat at Jody Maroni's Sausage Kingdom: The sausages and "Haute Dogs" wrapped in lettuce are your best choices here. All sausages except for the smoked chicken Cubana contain less than three grams of carbs.

KFC
★ | $

www.kfc.com

Thousands of restaurants throughout the United States and much of the world.

Claim to Fame: fried chicken

THE GOOD
Some KFC stores also house a Taco Bell in the same building (you can even order from both restaurants at the same drive-through window), which widens your low-carb options somewhat. Otherwise don't come to KFC if you don't love chicken. Even then, eating low-carb at KFC takes some willpower and planning.

THE BAD
Almost everything on the menu is high in carbohydrates, including *all* side dishes except the green beans. KFC's famous cole slaw, while always a consumer favorite, packs twenty-two grams of carbohydrates in a 4.5-ounce serving. Even with a fiber count of three grams, this still makes an effective carb count of about nineteen grams. Unless you have the discipline to remove the skin and breading, chicken breasts make the worst poultry choice. A traditional recipe chicken breast contains eleven grams of carbs. Make that extra-crispy style, and the count goes up to nineteen grams. A "hot and spicy" chicken breast has twenty grams of carbs.

THE UGLY
Surprisingly, one of the worst high-carb offenders at KFC—aside from potatoes and beans—are the BBQ beans. A single serving contains 38 net carbs.

The Best Things to Eat at KFC: At zero carbs, a chicken

breast with skin and breading removed is the best thing to eat at KFC. If you don't have the willpower to remove skin and breading, ordering Original Recipe as opposed to Extra Crispy or Hot and Spicy style chicken will consistently save you carbs at KFC, as the counts in the chart below illustrate.

	Original Recipe	Extra Crispy	Hot and Spicy
Breast	11g	19g	20g
Drumstick	4g	5g	4g
Thigh	12g	12g	14g
Wing	5g	10g	19g

KRYSTAL
★ | $
www.krystal.com

Over 420 restaurants in twelve states, with concentrations in the south.

Claim to Fame: tiny hamburgers served on dinner rolls

THE GOOD
The fillings of Krystal's burgers and breakfast sandwiches have minimal carbs.

THE BAD
The sandwiches are tiny, especially when you just want the fillings.

THE UGLY
Don't go near the fries, with or without chili. The lemon ice box pie will set your diet back by thirty-nine net carb grams and there are twenty-nine grams in a fried apple turnover.

The Best Things to Eat at Krystal: For zero to one carb, burgers without the buns are best, but the burgers here are so small this doesn't give you a whole lot of volume. So small are Krystal burgers, you can almost get away with eating the bread, if you can manage to only eat one. A regular-sized Krystal or bacon Krystal burger contains fourteen net carb grams, fifteen in a single cheese Krystal burger. The chicken bites salad does contain breaded fried chicken, but still retains a modest carb count of eight net carbs. A cup of Krystal's chili weighs in with an effective carb count of fifteen grams.

Breakfast: Forget about sandwiches and complete meals and go straight to the â la carte menu where you can get eggs cooked the way you like them, bacon, and Jimmy Dean sausage—all virtually carb-free.

LONG JOHN SILVER'S
★ | $

www.longjohnsilvers.com
Over 1,400 restaurants nationwide.
Claim to Fame: seafood/fish and chips

THE GOOD
At zero carbs, you can't do any better than the baked cod. That said, the rest of Long John Silver's menu is pretty bleak from a low-carb standpoint. So you'll find something to eat, just not a wide variety.

THE BAD
Aside from the baked cod, all the fish, shrimp, clams, and chicken at Long John Silver's are battered and fried. If you have the discipline to remove the breading, these items will have a negligible carb count. Even a single tiny hushpuppy packs nine grams.

THE UGLY
Beware of the clam chowder, as it contains twenty-three grams of carbs. An order of rice contains thirty-four grams of carbs. It goes without saying Long John's pies are off limits.

The Best Things to Eat at Long John Silver's: With only 4.5 grams of fat and no carbs, the baked cod is by far the healthiest item to order at Long John Silver's. Side dishes are questionable, depending on which diet you are following. An order of cole slaw has an effective carb count of eleven. Ditto a corn cobette. We can only hope this chain will add more low-carb items in the future.

MCDONALD'S
★★ | $
www.mcdonalds.com
Huge megachain found around the world.
Claim to Fame: hamburgers

THE GOOD
McDonald's has added some decent low-carb salads and recently started offering bunless sandwiches, served with a knife and fork.

THE BAD
Avoid topping your salad with butter garlic croutons and you'll save yourself eight grams of carbs. While McDonald's cobb salad (with or without chicken) makes a good low-carb meal, avoid the Newman's Own cobb dressing usually served with them—a two ounce serving contains nine carb grams. Even without the bun, the filet of fish sandwich runs eleven carb grams, a McChicken sandwich has fourteen grams, and a crispy chicken sandwich fifteen grams. There are better choices here.

THE UGLY
Tempting as they may be, a small bag of French fries carries an effective carb count of twenty-four grams. Forget about shakes. A small twelve-ounce shake packs twenty-two carb grams; super-size it, and that number balloons to 178 grams. Of course, all desserts are off limits.

The Best Things to Eat at McDonalds: For the healthiest choices, go straight to the salads. A California cobb salad (without chicken) has an effective carb count of just four grams. A grilled chicken bacon ranch salad, a grilled chicken cobb salad, or a grilled chicken Caesar salad each contain only six net carb grams. McDonald's serves

Newman's Own salad dressings. Best bets are the creamy Caesar, low-fat Balsamic, or ranch flavors, at four grams per serving.

Low-carbers can get any McDonald's sandwiches served on a bed of whole leaf lettuce with a knife and fork instead of on a bun. The following carb counts are given for the sandwiches with McDonald's usual fixings, but without bread. In some cases, you can lower the carb counts further by eliminating certain ingredients, such as ketchup or special sauce.

A Chicken McGrill contains only four carb grams. A Big N' Tasty burger has five grams; a regular McDonald's hamburger, a Big N' Tasty with cheese, or a Quarter Pounder with cheese all contain six net carbs; a regular cheeseburger or a Double Quarter Pounder with cheese have seven grams; and a Big Mac or Hot and Spicy McChicken both weigh in at ten grams.

Breakfast: Forget sandwiches or meals and order your McDonald's breakfast a la carte where you can fill up on scrambled eggs (one carb gram per two eggs), bacon, and sausage (zero carbs).

PANDA EXPRESS
★★★ | $–$$
www.pandaexpress.com
More than 600 locations nationwide.
Claim to Fame: Chinese fast food

THE GOOD
Surprisingly, there's a lot for low-carb dieters to eat at Panda Express—meats, seafood, and vegetables in tasty Chinese sauces.

THE BAD
Avoid the sweet and sour dishes—a four-ounce serving of chicken will cost you twenty-eight grams of carbs, seventeen grams for sweet and sour pork. The fried shrimp at twenty-eight grams for six pieces are also off limits. Skip the egg rolls, too; the chicken version contains twenty-one grams, and the veggie spring roll has fourteen grams.

THE UGLY
At fifty carbs per 5.5-ounce serving, the orange chicken will break the carb bank. Dinners here usually come with rice or chow mein noodles. An eight-ounce serving of steamed rice contains seventy-four grams of carbs; sixty-one grams for vegetable fried rice; and forty-eight grams for vegetable chow mein. Luckily, you can choose to forego the starches and get an order of mixed veggies and tofu instead.

The Best Things to Eat at Panda Express: A 5.5-ounce serving of chicken with mushrooms has an effective carb count of just five grams. Second best is Mandarin chicken with six net carbs, followed by black pepper chicken at seven grams and chicken with string beans for nine grams. Beef lovers can chow down on beef with broccoli for eight net carbs or beef with string beans for nine grams. Veggie lovers will appreciate the mixed vegetables with tofu at seven net grams of carbohydrates or the string beans with fried tofu for eight grams. Substitute an order of vegetables with tofu for the usual high-starch rice and chow mein noodles that usually come with combo dinners.

PAPA MURPHY'S
★★ | $–$$
www.papamurphys.com
Over 800 restaurants in twenty-three states.
Claim to Fame: take-and-bake pizza

THE GOOD
Low-carbers—especially those on maintenance—will love Papa Murphy's new thin crust deLITE pizza, which contains fewer than half the carbohydrates and almost half the calories of Papa Murphy's standard bake-at-home pizzas.

THE BAD
An order of two cheesy bread sticks will cost you twenty-three carb grams. Eating a slice of regular-crust Papa Murphy's pizza will hurt your diet to the tune of about thirty carbs per slice.

THE UGLY
You might think you'd be safe from desserts at a take-and-bake pizza shop, but you'd be wrong. Papa Murphy's also makes dessert pizzas, at forty-four carbs per slice for cherry and forty-seven grams per slice for apple. They also offer chocolate chip cookie dough that you can take home and bake up hot cookies any time you want in the comfort of your own home. Don't do it! Two cookies contain thirty-four carb grams.

The Best Things to Eat at Papa Murphy's: For truly low-carb fare, look to Papa Murphy's salads. An individual-size Italian salad contains just four net carb grams, five net carbs for an individual garden salad, and seven net carbs for a club salad. Aside from salads, Papa Murphy's thin crust deLITE pizzas come in four varieties, each containing eleven carb grams per slice: thin crust veggie deLITE tops a thin, reduced-carb pizza crust with creamy garlic sauce and covers it with cheese, spinach, mushrooms, and Roma tomatoes; thin crust pepperoni deLITE features tomato sauce, a cheese blend, and Italian pepperoni; thin crust meat deLITE tops the crust with tomato sauce, cheese, and precooked Italian sausage and ground beef (precooking results in a leaner product); tomato sauce, and Papa Murphy's special cheese blend covers the thin crust cheese deLITE pizza. Of course, to reduce carbs further, you can always eat the low-carb pizza toppings and leave the crust behind.

QDOBA MEXICAN GRILL
★★★ | $
www.qdoba.com
In twenty-three states, with concentrations in the east.
Claim to Fame: Mexican food

THE GOOD
As all menu items at Qdoba are made to order, it's easy to get exactly what you want and leave off the foods you don't. Order your burrito with extra meat and cheese, no rice, or beans with a low-carb salsa, then toss the tortilla for a hearty meal with negligible carbs. You'll also find some great salad options.

THE BAD
Items like beans and rice add carbs to your count, but at least the beans are healthy, fiber-rich carbs that some diet plans encourage.

THE UGLY
Stay away from the nachos—the tortilla chips can add 40 or more carb grams to your daily count.

The Best Things to Eat at Qdoba: Qdoba serves a low-carb salad consisting of chicken, lettuce, picante ranch dressing, mild salsa, and cheese, which contains about nine grams of carbohydrates. Aside from that, it's difficult to give exact quotes for Qdoba food as it depends on how you order it. Mix and match low-carb burrito fillings like beef, chicken, cheese, lettuce, and salsas or hot sauces; just remember to leave the tortilla behind and eat the fillings and you'll stay well within your daily carb limit.

QUIZNOS SUB
★★★★ | $–$$
www.quiznos.com
Over 1,800 restaurants in forty-seven states and thirteen countries.

Claim to Fame: toasted sub sandwiches

THE GOOD
Quiznos recently introduced twenty-four new low-carb sandwiches, each containing fewer than ten grams net carbs. You can also get some good low-carb salads here. New promotional material proudly proclaims that Quiznos offers "more low-carb choices than anyone on the planet." A heavy statement to make, but the new flat-bread sandwiches do open the door to endless carb-legal sandwich combinations.

THE BAD
Eating the regular Quiznos bread will cost you thirty or more grams of carbs.

THE UGLY
Don't even consider ordering potato chips or Quiznos cookies, brownies, or bundt cakes.

The Best Things to Eat at Quiznos: Quiznos new low-carb sandwiches are served on low-carb flatbread instead of the usual sub roll. The sandwiches are still toasted and have the same great flavor as the originals, but without the carbohydrates. The following will give you net carb counts for sandwiches ordered without dressing (not all sandwiches are available at all Quiznos locations):

Chicken carbonara (5.8 net carbs), double cheese (6.4), bacon, lettuce, and tomato (6.7), honey bourbon chicken (6.9), tuna (7.2), beef and cheddar (7.2), honey mustard chicken with bacon (7.4), mesquite chicken with bacon (7.6), Black Angus steak (7.7), Sierra smoked turkey (7.9), pastrami (8.1), smoked turkey (8.3), oven roasted turkey (8.4), classic Italian (8.5), spicy Monterey club (8.6), meatball (9.0), classic club with bacon (9.1), Philly cheesesteak (9.5), turkey ranch and swiss (9.6), veggie (9.7), turkey lite (9.7), ham and swiss (9.7), Quiznos Traditional (9.9), honey bacon club (10.3).

If you want forego bread altogether, order a Quiznos salad (hold the croutons in all cases). For about four net carbs, you can get a side green salad or small Caesar salad. For main courses try the chicken Caesar or the turkey, ranch, and Swiss salad for about eight net carbs.

SCHLOTZSKY'S DELI
★★★★ | $–$$
www.schlotzskys.com

Over 560 restaurants in thirty-seven states and six countries.

Claim to Fame: sandwiches and deli food

THE GOOD
Any of Schlotzsky's dozen or more sandwiches are now available wrapped in a low-carb tortilla (seven grams net carbs) or served on a bed of lettuce. In addition, you'll find a number of low-carb, high-fiber salads, soups, and side dishes.

THE BAD
Don't even look at the carb-glutted dessert menu, which includes temptations like fresh baked cookies and creamy New York–style cheesecake. Eat any of the desserts and you'll be consuming between twenty to forty-six grams of carbs.

THE UGLY
Schlotzsky's famous bread is delicious but carb-loaded. A six-inch sourdough bun, dark rye bun, or sourdough pizza crust contains sixty-eight carb grams; jalapeno cheese or wheat bun has sixty-six grams.

The Best Things to Eat at Schlotzsky's Deli: For entrée salads, try the chicken Caesar (two grams net carbs), Greek salad (six net carbs) Chinese chicken salad (eight carbs) or Smoked Turkey Chef's Salad (ten carbs). A regular order of chicken salad has just nine net carbs—eight for albacore tuna salad. Even the California pasta salad is a decent choice at nine carbs per five-ounce serving. Craving something hot and hearty? Try soups: Tuscan tomato basil soup has ten net carbs per cup serving; without rice, chicken gumbo weighs in at eleven net carbs; tortilla soup or gourmet vegetable beef contain twelve net carbs each; and minestrone or vegetarian vegetable have fourteen each.

Choices in the sandwich department are legion. Add seven net grams to the following carbs counts if you opt for tortilla-wrapped sandwiches instead of breadless versions. For just two grams of carbs, order a bunless albacore tuna melt, chicken breast, chicken club, Dijon chicken, pesto chicken, vegetable club, or western vegetable sandwich. For three grams, order a bunless small Schlotzsky's Original, fiesta chicken, Santa Fe chicken or roast beef sandwich. Four carbs will buy you a bunless small ham and cheese, smoked turkey breast, Philly, or turkey rueben. For six carbs, order a small bunless deluxe Schlotzsky's Original or corned beef reuben. The highest-carb sandwich on the entire menu is the Texas Schlotzsky's, at nine grams for a small breadless sandwich.

SBARRO
★★★ | $–$$
www.sbarro.com
Over 1,000 restaurants across the United States—often in shopping malls or airports.
Claim to Fame: Italian food, pasta, and pizza

THE GOOD
You'll find some tasty salads and usually a protein entrée or two at Sbarro.

THE BAD
The pizza here looks phenomenal—and of course they always have it prominently displayed. It doesn't matter, you can't get away from the tantalizing aroma anyway. Pasta fans will also have a lots of dishes they'll need to resist at Sbarro.

THE UGLY
An order of spaghetti with sauce comes with a side order of 110 net carb grams. A single, albeit large, slice of Sbarro's pizza will run you over eighty grams. Wow! A piece of chocolate cake only carries, in comparison, a moderate net carb count of fifty-eight grams.

The Best Things to Eat at Sbarro: Salads and chicken are the best low-carb things to order at Sbarro. For just four net carbs you can get a Greek salad, four for a mixed garden salad, five for a Caesar salad, and seven net carbs for a serving of cucumber and tomato salad or string bean and tomato salad. You can also get a side dish of mixed vegetables that includes zucchini, yellow squash, broccoli florets, and baby carrots cooked with lightly seasoned oil for about ten net carbs.

For entrées choose the six net carb chicken Francese, a sautéed, egg-battered chicken breast in a lemon sauce with sliced mushrooms and parsley, or the seven net carb chicken Vesuvio, sautéed egg-battered chicken breast with mushroom sauce and seasoned mushrooms. Even though it is lightly breaded, the chicken Parmigiana—topped with mozzarella cheese and tomato sauce—contains only fourteen net carb grams. All of these entrées typically come with pasta or potatoes. Skip the starch and get veggies or salad instead.

TACO BELL
★★ | $
www.tacobell.com
Thousands of restaurants throughout the United States and Canada, with limited international locations.
Claim to Fame: Mexican fast food

THE GOOD
There's a lot for low-carbers to eat at Taco Bell, providing you have the discipline to toss the tortillas and taco shells. That's really the only secret you need to know to eat at Mexican restaurants—eat the filling, leave the carbs behind. Also know that some KFC restaurants offer a limited Taco Bell menu.

THE BAD
Depending on the low-carb plan you follow, you may or may not have to hold the beans on your Taco Bell menu choices. A regular sized order of pintos and cheese runs fourteen grams of net carbs.

THE UGLY
The hard shell on Taco Bell's regular-style taco contains a modest ten carb grams. However, leaving the tortilla on your soft taco will cost you eighteen grams of carbs and a burrito-sized tortilla weighs in at a whopping thirty-five grams. Don't think you can get away with cheating on your taco salad either—the fried tortilla "bowl" contains about forty grams of carbs. Steer clear of the cinnamon twists, Taco Bell's sweet dough dessert that packs twenty-eight grams of carbs per serving.

The Best Things to Eat at Taco Bell: From a low-carb perspective, it doesn't much matter if you order from Taco Bell's regular or "al fresco" style menu. The latter items are generally lighter and lower in calories, but the extras contained in the regular versions like sour cream or extra cheese are perfectly legal on most low-carb plans. Take away the tortillas and any of Taco Bell's ground beef, steak, or chicken tacos have only one to three grams of carbs. Wrapless "supreme" steak or chicken chalupas have only three grams of carbs; five for beef. In the salad category, the regular-style taco salad, without the fried tortilla shell, weighs in at thirty-three grams, although its twelve grams of fiber brings the effective carb count down to twenty-one. Skip the beans in your taco salad and the net carb count lowers to ten grams.

If you happen to be dining at a Taco Bell Express (smaller restaurants found in airports, stores, and shopping malls) you can order the express taco salad with chips. Pass on the chips and you'll consume twenty-four net carbs. Skip the chips and beans and the effective carb count lowers to eight.

TOGOS
★★ | $–$$
www.togos.com
Over 400 restaurants in nineteen states, with concentrations in the west.
Claim to Fame: submarine sandwiches

THE GOOD
The salads at Togo's are the low-carb meal of choice.

THE BAD
A single serving of potato salad will set you back twenty-one carb grams, twenty-two for a small baked potato. A seemingly innocent cup of chicken noodle soup contains eighteen not-so-innocent carb grams.

THE UGLY
Eating the bread on a small sub can cost you thirty-five carb grams or more. Stay away from the taco salad, as it contains sixty-five net carbs, forty-one for the oriental chicken salad.

The Best Things to Eat at Togo's: The chicken Caesar salad contains ten net carbs, but you can reduce that number to about two by leaving the croutons off. Skip the croutons on the farmer's market salad and you can shave its thirteen net carbs down to about four. Because of its grapes, the Napa spinach salad contains fifteen net carbs, but if your plan allows fruit, it's a delicious and healthy alternative.

A few of Togo's soups will fit into some low-carb plans. A small broccoli cheese soup has nine net carbs, ten for a small cup of chili, and twelve for turkey pot pie soup.

WENDY'S
★★★ | $
www.wendys.com
Wendy's has 6,500 restaurants in the United States, Canada, and internationally.
Claim to Fame: burgers

THE GOOD
Wendy's has a nice selection of salad options, and like most burger joints, Wendy's offers all their sandwiches without the bread. As I write this, Wendy's is developing a new low-carb menu, although it won't be available until after this book goes to print. Check Wendy's Web site for updates.

THE BAD
As usual, the bread will break your carb allowance bank: thirty-one carb grams per regular bun or thirty-eight for a kaiser roll. A small eight-ounce order of Wendy's chili packs sixteen net carbs. Even without the chips, Wendy's taco salad still contains twenty-nine grams of carbs.

THE UGLY
Wendy's famous Frosty dessert will really cost you—fifty-six carb grams per small twelve-ounce cup. Of course, you don't need me to tell you not to order the fries—a medium order also has fifty-six grams. Avoid the chicken strips, too; three strips contain thirty-three carb grams.

The Best Things to Eat at Wendys: For about six carbs, you can have a Wendy's classic single, double, or triple hamburger, or grilled chicken sandwich; just ask servers to withhold the bread and request a fork and knife. Feel free to add bacon for no additional carbs; cheese is less than one gram per slice. Forget the dressings that normally come with Wendy's Garden Sensations salads; most are unnecessarily high in carbs (even the usually low ranch dressing has five grams). Instead order the Caesar dressing (less than one gram) or the blue cheese (three grams). At nine carbs, plan on passing on the croutons. Follow this advice and the spinach chicken salad (without dressing) and the chicken BLT salad have just six net carbs. Without the honey-roasted pecans and house vinaigrette, the spring mix salad has an effective carb count of seven grams. Leave off the crispy rice noodles and oriental sesame dressing, and Wendy's Mandarin chicken salad weighs in at fourteen net carbs.

WHATABURGER
★★★ | $$$
www.whataburger.com
Hundreds of restaurants in nine south and southwestern
states and one Mexico location.
Claim to Fame: burgers

THE GOOD

Even though this is a quick service restaurant (the
proper industry term for fast food), Whataburger is
committed to building a custom burger that meets
your taste and dietary needs. Just tell them what you
want (or don't want) and they'll make it for you.

THE BAD

A small-size fries carries an effective carb count of
thirty grams—the same amount as a serving of apple
pie. At breakfast, don't let the biscuits tempt you.
Despite their light and fluffy appearance, a single
buttermilk biscuit packs in thirty-four grams of net
carbs.

THE UGLY

The shakes are loaded with carbs—over one hundred
for a small serving. The breakfast pancakes can also
wreak major damage with 114 net carb grams—and
that's before you add syrup!

The Best Things to Eat at Whataburger: Without the
bun, a double meat Whataburger or a Whataburger with
bacon and cheese contain just three grams of net carbs
each. Make that a bunless grilled chicken sandwich, and
it will cost you nine net carbs. For about six grams of net
carbs, you can get a garden salad with cheese and bacon.

WHITE CASTLE
★ | $

www.whitecastle.com

Almost 400 restaurants, with concentrations in the east and midwest.

Claim to Fame: tiny hamburgers served on dinner rolls

THE GOOD

The fillings of these sandwiches, burgers, have zero carbs.

THE BAD

The burgers here are so tiny, you'd have to eat a lot of them in order not to feel hungry.

THE UGLY

All side dishes are high-carb and off limits: French fries, onions rings, and breaded, fried cheese sticks.

The Best Things to Eat at White Castle: For less than one carb, burgers without the buns are best, but they don't give you a lot of food. The sandwiches here are so tiny, you can almost get away with eating the bread—if you can limit how many you eat. A regular-sized White Castle hamburger, cheeseburger, or bacon cheeseburger (with bread) contains nine net carbs each. And if you have to eat fries, while it is ill-advised, this is the place to do it—a small order of French fries at White Castle weighs in at a modest thirteen grams of net carb grams.

WIENERSCHNITZEL

★ | $

www.wienerschnitzel.com

Over 300 restaurants in ten states, with concentrations in California, the northwest, the southwest, and Guam.

Claim to Fame: hot dogs

THE GOOD

If you enjoy a good dog, this is the place for you.

THE BAD

Everything here comes on bread, so be prepared to toss the bun. Low-carb side dishes are nonexistent. Stick to the hot dogs; for some reason, the bratwursts, Italian sausages, and Polish sausages have higher carb counts.

THE UGLY

A small order of fries will cost you twenty-eight grams of carbs. Make those chili cheese fries and the number rises to thirty-nine. Jalapeno poppers weigh in at thirty-seven grams and onion rings fifty-six.

The Best Things to Eat at Wienerschnitzel: As long as you don't eat the bun, you can have any of Wienerschnitzel's hot dogs—except the BBQ bacon dog—for under seven net carbs. Yes, that even includes the chili cheese dog. You can also order bunless burgers. The meat has zero carbs. Keep the fixings low-carb (that means no ketchup), and you've got nothing to worry about.

Casual Restaurants

BAKER'S SQUARE

★★★ | $$

www.bakerssquarerestaurants.com

Over 150 restaurants, with concentrations in California and the upper midwest.

Claim to Fame: pies/casual cuisine

THE GOOD

If you can resist the pies, there's lots to eat at Baker's Square, including great salads and meat dishes, as well as veggie side dishes and breakfast items.

THE BAD

Stay away from the appetizer menu; pretty much everything on it is breaded, fried, and high in carbs.

THE UGLY

Baker's Square is famous for its pies, and as soon as you enter the door, you'll be faced with a tempting, mouthwatering display of the carb-offensive desserts. Don't look! Even the sugar-free versions have substantial carbs due to the crust.

The Best Things to Eat at Baker's Square: The chef's salad gives you a nice variety of foods, including mixed greens topped with slow-roasted turkey breast, smoked ham, mozzarella and cheddar cheeses, sliced eggs, black olives, and tomatoes, for about twelve to fourteen grams of net carbs. In the same carb count range is the Cobb salad, always a low-carb favorite with a bed of greens topped with grilled chicken breast, avocado, cheddar cheese, bacon, tomatoes, and sliced egg. The grilled chicken breast salad contains avocado, cheddar cheese, black olives, and tomatoes on a bed of crisp lettuce for about ten to twelve grams of net carbs. The chicken (or turkey) Caesar salads are also good bets, especially if you leave off the croutons, which will save you about ten to twelve net carb grams, giving these a net carb count of about eight to ten grams.

With any of Baker's Square entrées, be sure to ask your server to hold the potatoes and substitute a low-carb side order of steamed veggies instead (about three to six net carbs, depending on the vegetable available). At zero carbs, your best bet is the sirloin steak. The ham steak, at about one carb gram, is a nice change of pace, as are the grilled portobello pork chops, containing about three to five grams of net carbs without gravy.

Breakfast: Like most coffee shops, you'll find lots of low- and no-carb breakfast items at Baker's Square. Keep in mind that breakfast fare is available all day at these restaurants, so don't limit yourself at lunch or dinnertime. Choose eggs, bacon, sausage, ham, or steak (no bread or hash browns, of course). Some Baker's Square omelets are also great choices. Order the ham and cheese, the sunrise omelet (mushrooms, green peppers, tomatoes, onions, and cheddar cheese), or the Baker's omelet (ham, mushrooms, green peppers, tomatoes, onions, and cheddar cheese) for a big breakfast with a small number of carbs—none should top ten net carbs.

BIG BOY
★★★ | $$
www.bigboy.com
Over 250 restaurants throughout the United States and
limited international locations.
Claim to Fame: burgers, coffee shop cuisine

THE GOOD
Like most coffee shops, low-carbers can find lots to
eat at Big Boy, although you'll have to skip their signature Big Boy hamburger—too much bread and the
Thousand Island-like sauce is high in sugar and carbs
too. Big Boy's salad bar makes it easy to eat your
veggies and limit carbs as you can pick and choose
exactly what you want to eat.

THE BAD
You'll find the usual high-carb culprits in the side
dish department—fries, mashed or baked potatoes,
onion rings, etc. Luckily, you can get low-carb veggies or a side order of tossed or Caesar salad.

THE UGLY
Forget milkshakes, hot fudge sundaes, or Big Boy's
seasonal favorite, fresh strawberry pie.

The Best Things to Eat at Big Boy: Most Big Boy
restaurants offer a fruit and salad bar that also includes
soups. Depending on the soup of the day, you start with
something hot and then custom-build your perfect low-
carb salad. You can also order a grilled chicken salad,
Caesar salad with or without chicken (skip the croutons),
or grilled chicken fajita salad—none should cost you more
than 10 net carbs and most of those come from healthy
vegetables. If a hot meal is more to your liking, try one of
Big Boy's burger or chicken platters, made with half-pound
of carb-free beef or a grilled boneless, skinless chicken

breast. Ask to substitute a tossed salad and steamed veggies for the fries and cole slaw that normally come with the meal (there is an additional charge). Other good ultra-low or no-carb choices at Big Boy include the sirloin steak, lemon baked cod, or mozzarella chicken, with low-carb side dishes like steamed veggies and green salad.

Breakfast: As long as you skip the hash browns and toast, choose from an assortment of breakfast meats, eggs, or hearty three-egg omelets stuffed with low-carb fillings like ham and cheese. Keep in mind that breakfast is served all day at Big Boy.

BOB EVANS/OWENS RESTAURANTS
★★★★ | $$
www.bobevans.com
(over 500 restaurants)Bob Evans are located primarily in
the east and midwest; Owens Restaurants are in Texas.
Claim to Fame: country cooking

THE GOOD
Any restaurant that bases its menu around American
homestyle foods can't be all bad, from the low-carb
perspective. Breakfast, lunch, or dinner, you'll find
lots of menu choices at these casual coffee shops,
which consistently serve good, quality meals. Mix
and match to your heart's delight from a wide variety
of meats, vegetables, and salads.

THE BAD
If the bread basket is your weakness, be sure to keep
it off the table as you'll find delicious rolls, biscuits,
and fruit and nut breads at Bob Evans. Think before
you eat. A single buttermilk biscuit will cost you thirty-six carb grams; a small slice of banana nut bread
forty-two grams. Also, avoid the wildfire barbecue
sauce or anything served with it—a single serving
packs twenty-two carb grams. Ditto the hot bacon
salad dressing—a 1.5-ounce serving will set you back
eighteen grams.

THE UGLY
At a gut-busting eighty-five grams of carbohydrates,
avoid the frosted cinnamon rolls at all costs. Of
course, everything on Bob's extremely tempting
dessert menu is a disaster for low-carbers. The worst
offender of all is the Reese's Peanut Butter Cup pie,
at 129 grams per slice.

The Best Things to Eat at Bob Evans: Mix and match

meats and low-carb side dishes to create your perfect meal. Good choices in the meat department include the T-bone steak, pork chops, grilled chicken, roast turkey, grilled catfish, and grilled salmon. Pair any of these no- and ultra low-carb entrées with a side salad (without croutons) for just five carbs; broccoli florets or green beans with ham for just eight healthy grams. The salad menu holds several filling options: the country spinach salad with grilled chicken, for eleven grams; Frisco salad with grilled chicken, for thirteen; Cobb salad, for fourteen; or the raspberry grilled chicken salad, for eighteen. For the salad dressings, ranch is best, with a 1.5-ounce serving containing just one carb gram, followed by lite ranch at two, blue cheese at three, and lite Italian at four.

Breakfast: Bob Evans conveniently offers two low-carb breakfast plates; each comes with three eggs and either one or two orders of breakfast meats (bacon, sausage links, or patties). That's it, all protein, no high-carb sides. You can also get cholesterol-free Egg Beaters for just two carbs per serving. A ham, sausage, and/or cheese omelet has zero carbs. Other satisfying choices are the border omelet (with sausage, veggies, ranchero sauce, and sour cream) or the farmer's market omelet (sausage, ham, bacon, veggies, and hollandaise sauce), for three grams, or the garden harvest omelet (veggies, cheese, and hollandaise sauce), for four. Like cereal? A bowl of plain oatmeal contains just six net carbs.

BONANZA/PONDEROSA
★★★★★ | $–$$
www.bonanzarestaurants.com
Located throughout the eastern half of the United States.
Claim to Fame: reasonably priced steaks

THE GOOD
These two family steakhouse chains, while acquired
by the same company, retain their unique names.
The menu offerings, however, are identical. That's
good news for low-carb dieters who can get grilled-
to-order steaks accompanied by a huge buffet of
salads and side dish options. While you will need
to exercise some restraint when it comes to volume,
the serve-yourself buffet does allow you to choose
exactly the foods that fit your diet.

THE BAD
Along with healthy low-carb offerings like green
salads and steamed vegetables, you'll find high-carb
foods throughout the all-you-can-eat food bar. Avoid
starches like breads, pastas, and potatoes, and stick to
the veggies your low-carb plan allows.

THE UGLY
The unlimited food bar also includes desserts. Avoid
these dietary sirens beckoning you to sabotage your
diet. There are plenty of legal low-carb choices at
this restaurant to keep you from straying from the
program.

The Best Things to Eat at Bonanza/Ponderosa: You'll
find lots of no carb entrée choices here like steaks,
prime rib, grilled chicken, grilled shrimp, or salmon. All
have virtually no carbs. Since the items on the food bar
change, we're unable to make specific side dish recommendations. Stick to what you know works: green salads,

low-carb fiber-filled veggies like green beans, broccoli, cauliflower, etc.

Breakfast: Some locations offer weekend all-you-can-eat breakfast buffets. Start your day the low-carb way by chowing down on eggs, omelets, bacon, ham, and sausage. Eat a late breakfast and you won't need lunch!

CARROWS
★★★ | $$–$$$
www.carrows.com
Over 130 restaurants in six states; concentrations in California, also Washington, Oregon, Nevada, and Texas.
Claim to Fame: casual coffee shop/American food

THE GOOD
Like most coffee shops, you can find a nice selection of salads and protein entrées at Carrows.

THE BAD
Like most coffee shops, you can also find a huge selection of high-carb foods like fries, batter-fried meats and veggies, and other off-limits items.

THE UGLY
Carrows serves sweet milkshakes and malts, decadent desserts like mile-high chocolate cake, and some sweet decadent breakfast items like cinnamon French toast or waffles covered in syrup or strawberries and whipped cream. Low-carbers need to avoid them all!

The Best Things to Eat at Carrows: Order entrées with a small green salad (hold the croutons) and steamed vegetables, about four to six net carbs each. For zero carbs, choose from a variety of grilled-to-order steaks, prime rib (after 4 P.M.), blackened or grilled Norwegian salmon or mahi-mahi, or Carrows blackened blue chicken—a spicy, blackened chicken breast topped with bleu cheese butter and crumbled bacon. Carrow's also offers a Caesar salad or grilled chicken caesar salad for about six to seven net carbs without croutons and a Cobb salad for about twelve to fourteen grams of net carbs.

Breakfast: In addition to the usual array of carbless breakfast items like eggs, bacon, sausage, and ham, you can build your own three-egg omelet at Carrows or choose several good low-carb combinations right off the menu. The sunrise surprise omelet fills three eggs with ham, bacon, onions, and red and green bell peppers and tops it all with melted cheddar cheese and sour cream sauce. The Californian omelet combines Jack cheese, Roma tomatoes, olives, and bacon. Carrows Greek veggie omelet folds three eggs over sautéed artichokes, red onions, Roma tomatoes, mushrooms, and fresh chopped basil with feta and cream cheese. These omelets should run about six to eight net carbs each. At about two grams, the carb count on the ham and cheese omelet is even lower.

COCO'S BAKERY RESTAURANT
★★★ | $$–$$$
www.cocosbakery.com
Nearly 500 restaurants in four states, concentrated in California; also, Washington, Nevada, Arizona, and Colorado, with limited international locations.

Claim to Fame: casual American food with in-store bakeries

THE GOOD
Like most coffee shops, Coco's offers a respectable selection of meats and salads.

THE BAD
Most of the menu, and most of the dish combinations on the menu, contain high-carb foods. Be sure to substitute for potatoes, rice, or pastas.

THE UGLY
Part of Coco's name is "bakery" and that means lots of tempting, freshly baked pies, biscuits, muffins, and more. Even the sugar-free pies contain substantial carbs—especially in their crusts. Some of the breakfasts are unusually decadent as well—strawberry stuffed French toast, Belgian waffles, and cinnamon roll French toast.

The Best Things to Eat at Coco's: Of course, Coco's offers a Caesar salad or a grilled chicken Caesar salad, about six to seven net carbs without croutons; and a Cobb salad for about twelve to fourteen grams of net carbs. A bit more unique is their Mediterranean chopped salad, which blends romaine lettuce, turkey, Roma tomato, red onion, cucumbers, and chopped egg, topped off with crumbled feta cheese. Ask your server to leave off the sweetly glazed walnuts and crispy, pizza dough wedges that normally come with salad and it should only cost you about eight to ten net carbs.

For zero-carb entrées choose the broiled Cajun fish or the T-Bone, Tuscan ribeye, or blue cheese topped sirloin steaks. Accessorize your entrée with a small garden salad (about 4–5 grams of net carbs without croutons) and the steamed vegetable of the day. You can also order a nice selection of bunless burgers and chicken sandwiches.

Breakfast: You can mix and match breakfast meats and eggs while skipping the usual bread and potato accompaniments for zero carbs, or order one of Coco's fluffy three-egg omelets. Build your own omelet filled with all your favorite low- and no-carb favorites—meats, cheese, and veggies. For about four grams of net carbs, start your day with a California omelet including creamy avocado, melted Monterey Jack cheese, and crispy bacon; or a vegetable omelet with broccoli, sautéed mushrooms, tomato, green onion, cheddar cheese, fresh salsa, and sour cream, for about eight to ten grams of net carbs.

CRACKER BARREL
★★★★ | $–$$
www.crackerbarrel.com
Nearly 500 restaurants in forty-one states.
Claim to Fame: country cooking

THE GOOD
With a basic American-style country cooking menu, you can choose from lots of meats, low-carb veggies and salads at Cracker Barrel, not to mention a wide variety of breakfast options.

THE BAD
You'll need to avoid the comfort food accompaniments like mashed potatoes, macaroni and cheese, dumplings, fried apples, and grits. Avoid anything breaded and fried, which isn't hard to do since there are so many other delicious options at Cracker Barrel.

THE UGLY
The homestyle desserts like cobblers, pies, ice creams, and apple dumplings are hard to resist; don't go anywhere near them as we're talking major refined carbs—figure at least sixty grams per serving on the low end.

The Best Things to Eat at Cracker Barrel: Pair the following no/low-carb meats—ribeye steak, roast beef, grilled chicken tenderloins, hickory smoked ham, grilled pork chops, spicy grilled catfish, or hamburger steak—with these low-carb sides: turnip greens or boiled cabbage (about three grams net carbs), green beans (four grams), or a side salad (about six grams net carbs without dressing or croutons). For about four carb grams, you can even get gravy on your meat or veggies. Cracker Barrel also offers some great entrée-sized salads including a chef's salad,

Cobb salad, turkey and cheese salad, mixed vegetable salad, and BLT salad. Pair any of these with low-carb dressings like blue cheese, ranch, or oil and vinegar and skip the croutons; none of these should set you back more than about fourteen net carbs.

Breakfast: Choose ham, bacon, sausage, and eggs à la carte, and you have a breakfast that's virtually free of temptation and carbohydrates.

DENNY'S
★★★★ | $$

www.dennys.com

Thousands of restaurants throughout the United States and internationally.

Claim to Fame: casual American food

THE GOOD

With basic fare like salads, burgers, and simple dinners, as well as breakfast served any time, low-carbers have always been able to find something to eat at Denny's, twenty-four hours a day, seven days a week. It's gotten even easier, however, since Denny's introduced their new Carb-Watch menu in April 2004.

THE BAD

Most Denny's meals—breakfast, lunch, and dinner—typically come with some sort of potatoes. Remember that a five-ounce order of fries comes with a price tag of fifty-seven grams of carbohydrates.

THE UGLY

At Denny's, you'll have to navigate around the usual culprits that lurk in most American restaurants. Try not to look at the tempting pies and desserts prominently displayed in showcases, on the menu, and in table-top marketing pieces. The worst offender of all is Denny's brownie a la mode. This delicious little diet-killer weighs in at a waist-expanding forty-seven grams of carbs. Keep in mind that a baked potato with skin is no better, with an effective carb count of forty-six grams.

The Best Things to Eat at Dennys: An order of nine buffalo wings has just eleven grams of carbs. The wings come accompanied by celery sticks and blue cheese dressing. While you'll find this offered on Denny's appetizer menu, it makes a satisfying low-carb dinner choice.

All of Denny's Carb-Watch meals come with sliced tomatoes. Lunch and dinner Carb-Watch offerings also include green beans. Side dishes are reflected in the following net carb counts.

For lunch, try a Carb-Watch burger. For ten net carb grams, you get a hamburger patty with two slices of Swiss cheese, garlic sautéed mushrooms, onions, and diced tomatoes, and topped with shredded cheddar cheese. Or try a Carb-Watch grilled chicken salad—grilled chicken breast sliced and served atop mixed greens with tomato, cucumber, red onions, and cheddar cheese, for six net carbs.

The Carb-Watch T-bone or sirloin steak dinner meals at Denny's contain just five grams of net carbs; six grams for Carb-Watch grilled chicken dinner; and eight grams for Denny's Carb-Watch roast turkey dinner.

Breakfast: For breakfast, try the Carb-Watch ham and cheddar omelet for seven grams net carbs; the ultimate Carb-Watch omelet for nine grams net carbs; or the Carb-Watch two-egg and three-meat breakfast, consisting of two eggs, two bacon strips, two sausage links, and a slice of grilled ham, served with sliced tomatoes, for just nine grams net carbs.

FUDDRUCKERS
★★★ | $–$$
www.fuddruckers.com
Over 220 restaurants in thirty states, Washington, D.C., and Puerto Rico.
Claim to Fame: burgers

THE GOOD
Company spokesperson J. Miller says the company has been amazed at how many requests they are getting for bunless burgers, and Fuddruckers is happy to comply. These are some of the best-tasting burgers in the country and they're just as tasty without the carb-filled bread; plus, Fuddruckers has just started a special new low-carb menu at most locations.

THE BAD
Leave the bread on and you'll consume thirty-five or more grams of carbohydrates.

THE UGLY
Forget about the baked or fried potatoes, baked beans, cole slaw, and chili cheese fries. Stick with meats and salads.

The Best Things to Eat at Fuddruckers: Fuddruckers burgers come in sizes to match every appetite: a third of a pound, half-pound, three-quarter pound, and one pound. You can also get turkey or ostrich (yes, ostrich) burgers in the one-third and two-thirds of a pound. Dress up your burger with no-carb toppings like bacon or your favorite cheeses. You can spend three to six grams of your daily carb gram allotment for your favorite accompaniments like lettuce, tomato, guacamole, grilled or raw onions, and/or grilled mushrooms or portobello mushrooms. Salad lovers can order a meal-sized Caesar salad, with or without grilled chicken or blackened ribeye steak. As long as you skip the croutons, none of the Caesar salads should run over twelve net carbs.

Most Fuddruckers also serve a low-carb menu that consists of grilled lemon pepper chicken breasts and a ten-ounce ribeye steak for about one carb; a two-thirds of a pound chopped steak topped with grilled onions and mushrooms, for about five to six grams of carbs; and a portobello melt—consisting of fresh ground beef over a portobello mushroom, blanketed in melted Swiss cheese—for about three to four carbs. Each of these entrées come, with a small garden salad (about four net carbs without croutons) and a low-carb steamed vegetable. While veggie choices change with market availability, you'll usually be safe budgeting between four to six net carbs for this side dish.

FURR'S CAFETERIA
★★★★ | $–$$
www.furrs.net
Over fifty restaurants in six southwest and midwest states, concentrated in Texas.
Claim to Fame: cafeteria

THE GOOD
Cafeterias are handy places for low-carbers in that they let you pick and choose from various menu items to create a perfect overall meal of just the food you like, or the foods that best fit within your diet plan. Most Furr's offer an all-you-can-eat pricing structure or a pay-by-the-item option. Survey the day's offerings for what will work best for you.

THE BAD
There are high-carb side dishes and breaded fried entrées you'll need to avoid.

THE UGLY
Bypass the dessert section. Luckily, it's not hard to do as there are always so many other good low-carb offerings here.

The Best Things to Eat at Furr's Cafeteria: The menu changes daily, so not all the low-carb items listed will be available at all times or in all locations. That said, you can always find green salads and low-carb steamed vegetable side dishes at Furr's. For no- and nearly no-carb entrées, choose from among baked or grilled fish, carved turkey or roast beef, rotisserie-style chicken, and liver and onions. The exact carb counts you consume will depend on the items you choose.

GOLDEN CORRAL
★★★★★ | $–$$
www.goldencorral.com
Over 470 restaurants throughout the United States.
Claim to Fame: reasonably priced steaks

THE GOOD
Any restaurant that serves grilled-to-order steaks will earn high marks in most low-carbers' opinions. Golden Corral does even more. You'll also find a large variety of carb-friendly salads, vegetables, side dishes, and yes—gasp!—even desserts!

THE BAD
The all-you-can-eat buffet that accompanies the steaks, while laden with high-carb diet busters, still contains enough sensible choices to make this a no-brainer when deciding what to eat—just avoid sugars and starches. The more important issue is deciding how much to eat, as the bottomless plates at Golden Corral make it easy to overindulge. At breakfast, avoid the corned beef hash (a single cup serving carries twenty-two carb grams) and the creamed chipped beef (nine grams per half-cup).

THE UGLY
Golden Corral gives low-carbers several sugar-free dessert choices, but stay away from their real sugar counterparts. A serving of carrot cake contains fifty-two grams of carbs; a single yeast dinner roll packs in forty-two carbs. Worst of all is the banana pudding, at seventy grams of carbs. And that's for only a half-cup!

The Best Things to Eat at Golden Corral: For zero, as in nada, zilch, carbs choose the sirloin steak, steakburgers, roast beef, pork chops, pork loin, salmon, or Cajun whitefish. For a single carb gram, chow down on rotisserie chicken, ham, turkey, or steamed whitefish. For side dishes, have some fresh steamed zucchini or cabbage for one carb gram, steamed cauliflower for two, squash medley for three, spinach, green and yellow beans, or Southern-style cabbage for four carbs. For just five grams, you can have steamed broccoli or half a cup of vegetable trio, while an order of green beans will cost you six carbs. For soups, try the chicken gumbo with an effective carb count of nine, the chicken noodle soup for eleven net carbs, or the broccoli cheese soup for eighteen. In addition to tossed green salad with low-carb dressings like creamy Caesar or oil and vinegar, check out Golden Corral's marinated vegetable salad (five grams per half cup); marinated mushrooms (six grams per half cup) and tuna salad (eight grams per half cup).

For dessert, you can order sugar-free red Jell-O for zero carbs. A half-cup serving of no-sugar-added chocolate pudding carries an effective carb count of fifteen. In the bakery department, a single sugar-free chocolate chip cookie or oatmeal bar will cost you about eleven net carbs.

Breakfast: Some Golden Corral restaurants offer an all-you-can-eat breakfast buffet that lets you build your own virtually carb-free meal with eggs, bacon, and sausage. If you leave the English muffin behind, you can even get eggs Benedict for about five carb grams.

HOMETOWN BUFFET/COUNTRY BUFFET/OLD COUNTRY BUFFET

★★★★★ | $–$$

www.hometownbuffet.com

There are 350 restaurants in thirty-eight states. Hometown Buffet is concentrated on the West Coast; Old Country Buffet is concentrated in the midwest and on the East Coast.

Claim to Fame: all-you-can-eat country cooking

THE GOOD

These low-cost buffets change their offerings daily, but low-carbers can rest assured they will always have a large number of food choices. The menu here is based on good old American food and lots of it—meats, vegetables, and salads.

THE BAD

To get to the good low-carb items, you'll have to navigate through at least three times as many high-carb, off-limits foods. Know what you are and aren't allowed and stick to your plan.

THE UGLY

Don't get anywhere near the all-you-can-eat desserts. This is the biggest high-carb stumbling block many people face at buffets. Don't even look. Fill up on the dinner, go back for a second helping of salad, fish, chicken, or beef, just avoid the sugar, and you'll be fine.

The Best Things to Eat at Hometown Buffet/Country Buffet/Old Country Buffet: It's difficult to make specific recommendations as the daily offerings at these buffets change constantly and not all items may be available at all locations at all times. That said, you can always find plenty to eat. Mix and match between baked chicken or fish, hot wings, sausage and sauerkraut, roast beef, roast turkey, peppered pork loin, and salmon filet. Choose low-carb side dishes like green beans, sautéed zucchini, spring greens—five net carb grams or less each.

Breakfast: Some buffet locations offer Saturday and Sunday breakfasts. What a great way to start a weekend day. Build your breakfast from popular no- and low-carb foods like eggs, ham, bacon, and sausage. The breakfast buffets even offer eggs benedict; just don't eat the bread. Some locations let you "build your own" Benedict, so you can leave off the English muffin and savor the Canadian bacon and poached eggs smothered in a decadent low-carb hollandaise sauce (about two grams per tablespoon).

IHOP (INTERNATIONAL HOUSE OF PANCAKES)
★★★★ | $$

www.ihop.com

Over 1,150 restaurants in forty-eight states and Canada.

Claim to Fame: pancakes and breakfast items

THE GOOD

With a little bit of creative menu selecting and substituting, this casual coffee shop offers a lot of low-carb options. There are several low-carb main course salads as well as entrées that can be accompanied by steamed veggies and salad instead of the usual fries or baked potatoes. You can get breakfast all day at IHOP, which substantially widens your dining options if you have the willpower to skip the pancakes and bread. Looking for something sweet? Order a plain omelet and top it with a little sugar-free pancake syrup.

THE BAD

As with most casual restaurants, your meal will regularly come with off-limit side dishes like potatoes or bread. Even IHOP's otherwise low-carb salads come with a nice warm slice of garlic cheese toast. Tell your server to leave it in the kitchen so you won't be tempted.

THE UGLY

The restaurant's namesake, pancakes, are definitely out of bounds for low-carbers. Don't even think about the syrups or sweet fruit toppings that get piled on top of them. Since IHOP offers so many other options, it's not too difficult to resist.

The Best Things to Eat at IHOP: For hearty anytime meals, try the Colorado omelet (bacon, pork sausage, shredded beef, ham, onions, green peppers, and cheddar cheese) for about five net carbs, the international omelet (ham, cheese, green peppers, onions, and salsa) for about eight net carbs, or build your own omelet with your choice of favorite low-carb fillings like meats, cheeses, and vegetables. Choose an entrée-sized southwestern fajita salad (skip the tortilla shell or cheese bread) or grilled chicken Caesar salad (skip the croutons and save about ten carb grams), for about ten net carbs. For hot entrées, try the herb-roasted chicken, grilled chicken breast, grilled fish, or T-bone steak. The meat has zero carbs and you can always get some type of low-carb steamed veggie here—selections change frequently.

JOHNNY ROCKETS
★★ | $–$$
www.johnnyrockets.com
Currently in twenty-eight states, primarily in the east and west; some international locations.
Claim to Fame: burgers in a 1950s-style diner setting

THE GOOD
You can ask for any Johnny Rockets sandwiches or burgers wrapped in lettuce instead of a bun, which will give you a tasty low-carb meal. There's a couple of good low-carb entrée-sized salads as well, and Johnny's chili is surprisingly ultra-low in carbs.

THE BAD
At this classic burger joint, most menu items come on bread, accompanied by fries or onion rings.

THE UGLY
Burgers are really only half of Johnny Rockets' claim to fame; their shakes and soda fountain treats make up the other half. Low-carbers should stay far away from this side of the menu.

The Best Things to Eat at Johnny Rockets: A chicken club salad, made with grilled chicken—as opposed to fried chicken tenders—carries an effective carb count of just seven grams. With just four net carbs, the small garden salad is the side dish of choice at Johnny Rockets. Aside from that, your options are to pick a burger or grilled chicken sandwich, topped with your favorite legal low-carb toppings, and ask for it lettuce-wrapped. Eat with a fork and knife like the civilized individual you are. It's easy to keep your carb count well under eight grams, even for burgers with all the fixings. Consider Johnny Rockets' chili. A bowl has an effective carb count of just six grams. Top your burger with a 2.5 ounce serving of chili for just one net carb.

MARIE CALLENDER'S
★★★★ | $–$$$
www.mariecallenders.com
Ninety-six restaurants in eleven western United States;
Utah locations do not offer alcoholic beverages.
Claim to Fame: pies/homestyle cooking

THE GOOD
The all-you-can-eat soup and salad bar makes it
easy to construct high-protein, low-carb salads just
the way you like them. Marie's also usually offers
a decent variety of steamed vegetables and always
serves fresh roasted turkey.

THE BAD
A lot of the straight-off-the-menu items that made
Marie's reputation are, unfortunately, high-carb.
Forget the pot pies or chicken-fried steak and stick to
grilled or roasted meats and veggies. Beware of high-
carb items on the salad bar like pastas and fruits.

THE UGLY
Marie's famous pies are diet-busters—flaky, floury
crusts filled with sugary sweet fillings.

The Best Things to Eat at Marie Callender's: Build your
own salad at the salad bar or order an entrée-sized Cobb
salad, Caesar salad (with or without grilled chicken or
roast turkey), or a Cabo San Lucas chicken salad (hold
the tortilla chips). None of these should run over twelve
net carb grams. For carb-free entrées, choose roast turkey,
lemon grilled chicken breasts, sirloin steak, grilled shrimp,
or baked or grilled fresh fish. Ask for low-carb steamed
veggies like asparagus, broccoli, cauliflower, or zucchini
on the side—about five to six net carbs per veggie.

Here's a tip! It's no longer on the menu, but you can
still order a plate of steamed vegetables covered with
melted cheese.

Breakfast: A few Marie Callender's serve breakfast. Order eggs, breakfast meats, and omelets made with low-carb veggies. We especially enjoy Marie's ham steak.

OLD SPAGHETTI FACTORY
★★★ | $–$$$
www.osf.com
Nearly forty restaurants in fifteen states, with concentrations in California and the northwest; some southwest, south, and midwest locations.
Claim to Fame: pasta

THE GOOD
Low-carbing pasta lovers on maintenance will love Old Spaghetti Factory's new reduced-carb pasta, with an effective carb count of nineteen grams per four ounce lunch serving (the same portion of regular pasta contains thirty-nine net carbs) or 28.5 grams per six-ounce dinner serving. Those in the induction or weight-loss phases of most low-carb diets will want to pass on the pasta, but it does offer a healthier, lower-carbohydrate way to indulge an occasional craving.

THE BAD
The bread comes to the table early and returns often at Old Spaghetti Factory—an endless supply of fragrant, hot-out-of-the-oven bread that magically keeps reappearing throughout the dinner. Sit as far away from the bread as possible to avoid temptation.

THE UGLY
The regular pastas start at sixty-one carbs per serving for fettuccine Alfredo and escalate to ninety-five grams for spaghetti with meatballs and tomato sauce, and 110 grams for spaghetti potpourri.

The Best Things to Eat at Old Spaghetti Factory: You can order baked chicken (zero to two carbs) or sausages (about one carb per sausage) a la carte. Another item that isn't always on the menu is steamed broccoli prepared just like Old Spaghetti Factory's pasta, with brown butter and mizithra cheese, but without the carbs of the pasta. Broccoli prepared this way is ultra-tasty and satisfying and contains about four to six net carbs. Unless you specify otherwise, the chicken Caesar salad comes with breaded, fried chicken. However, you can request grilled chicken instead of fried, creating a main dish salad that contains about seven to nine net carbs (without croutons). If you do need to splurge on pasta, order the reduced-carb versions. The lowest carb toppings are the Alfredo sauce, and brown butter and mizithra Cheese. All of Old Spaghetti Factory's salad dressings are two grams of carbs or less, except for Thousand Island and honey mustard.

PERKINS RESTAURANT AND BAKERY

★★★★ | $–$$

www.perkinsrestaurants.com

Over 475 restaurants in thirty-four states and parts of Canada.

Claim to Fame: home-style cooking

THE GOOD

An all-day breakfast menu plus good basic coffee-shop fare and creative salads give low-carbers lots of options when eating at Perkins.

THE BAD

As with most coffee shops, there are lots of fried, breaded menu items, as well as sweet and starchy offerings. Skip the appetizer, burger, and sandwich menus entirely and head for the dinner or breakfast choices instead.

THE UGLY

Many of Perkins's best low-carb salads come served in freshly baked crispy Italian bread bowls. Be sure to ask your server to bring yours on a plate instead. Perkins also has an in-house bakery that will try to tempt you with sweet, gooey treats. Luckily, there are lots of other great things to eat here to help you resist.

The Best Things to Eat at Perkins: From the dinner menu, choose grilled pork chops, top sirloin or New York strip steaks, grilled lemon pepper grouper, or oven-roasted chicken, for zero carbs. For side dishes, have a small green salad, cottage cheese, steamed broccoli, or green beans with bacon—about four to six net carbs each. The Greek spinach salad—spinach and lettuce with grilled lemon pepper chicken, red onions, black olives, tomatoes, cucumbers, red peppers, and feta cheese—is a great entrée salad choice. The remaining low-carb entrée salads all come in a fresh-baked edible bread bowl. Save yourself *beaucoups* temptation and make sure the bread bowl never sets down on your table when ordering the following high-fiber, low-carb salads: BLT chicken breast salad, chef salad, or lemon pepper chicken Caesar salad (save about ten carbs and hold the croutons). These salads should run in the ten to fourteen net carb range.

Breakfast: Breakfast at Perkins is served all day, so don't forget to look at this portion of the menu when making selections. In addition to the usual array of à la carte breakfast items like eggs, bacon, sausage, steak, or ham, Perkins offers some terrific omelets that also make satisfying low-carb lunches or dinners. Try the everything omelet (cheese, ham, mushrooms, green peppers, tomatoes, onions, and celery), the farmhouse garden omelet (broccoli florets, red peppers, mushrooms, and pepper Jack cheese with hollandaise sauce), country club omelet (roasted turkey breast, bacon, green onions, and tomatoes, with hollandaise sauce), or build your own omelet with the low-carb ingredients you love best.

PICCADILLY CAFETERIA
★★★★★ | $–$$
www.piccadilly.com
Over 130 restaurants, largely in the south and midwest.
Claim to Fame: all-you-can-eat cafeteria

THE GOOD
Here's one cafeteria that recognizes the importance of the low-carb market. As such, you can always find a large array of carb-friendly vegetables as well as lots of protein-filled main courses. Eating at Piccadilly is always a low-carb breeze. While menu offerings change daily, Piccadilly always offers at least four low-carb salads, side dishes, and entrées each and every day. In-store indicators make it easy to identify any menu items containing less than ten carb grams per serving.

THE BAD
You'll have to monitor your own portion control. The allure of all-you-can-eat food, even if it is low-carb food, can sabotage weight loss for some folks.

THE UGLY
While Piccadilly recognizes low-carbers, they also cater to a regular market, so avoid starches and especially desserts.

The Best Things to Eat at Piccadilly: For zero-carb entrées, choose unbreaded meats like roast beef, rotisserie or grilled chicken, roast turkey, marinated pork loin, steaks, or a variety of baked or Cajun-blackened fish. The stuffed catfish or basa have just eight carb grams each. For side dishes, you'll find lots of veggie choices including (approximate net carbs per half-cup serving): bacon-seasoned spinach, steamed cabbage with bacon, fresh broccoli, or buttered cauliflower, about three net carbs;

green beans, for about four net carbs; Brussels sprouts, Creole okra, mixed vegetables, or collard or turnip greens with diced turnips, about five net carbs. In addition to the usual low-carb green salad, you can also get cucumbers with sour cream (5 net carbs), asparagus and tomato salad (eight), cauliflower salad (seven), Italian cole slaw (three), kosher cole slaw (five), or cucumber and celery salad (eight). Don't overlook Piccadilly's soups, either. A bowl of chicken or chicken and sausage gumbo has just nine net carb grams, providing you leave out the rice. You can even end your Piccadilly meal on a sweet note with a bowl of sugar-free Jell-O, for zero carbs.

Breakfast: Most Piccadilly locations offer all-you-can-eat breakfast buffets on weekends. Start your day by constructing your personal, perfect low- or no-carb breakfast with eggs, bacon, sausage, ham, and more.

PIZZA HUT
★★ | $–$$
www.pizzahut.com
Thousands of restaurants across the United States and in ninety international countries.
Claim to Fame: pizza

THE GOOD
Even if you lack the discipline to eat only the pizza toppings and leave the crust, you can still find some good things to eat at Pizza Hut restaurants, although the fare at the Pizza Hut Express restaurants, which caters primarily to the delivery or take-out trade, is pretty bleak from a low-carb perspective.

THE BAD
Some—although not all—Pizza Huts offer pastas, which low-carb dieters should definitely avoid. No matter what, you'll always have to contend with the temptation of freshly baked pizza dough. Although not ultra-high in carbs, two fried mozzarella sticks contain thirteen grams of carbs due to their breading.

THE UGLY
With every single breadstick you consume at Pizza Hut, you'll also consume twenty grams of carbs. Three ounces of breadstick dipping sauce will add another eleven grams. Stay away from Thousand Island salad dressing; it contains eleven carb grams per two tablespoons. All of the desserts fall into the "coyote ugly" category in regard to carbs. Two pieces of cinnamon sticks pack twenty-seven grams of carbs. Two ounces of the White Icing dipping sauce will skyrocket your insulin levels to the tune of forty-six carb grams! A single slice of Pizza Hut's dessert pizzas will cost your carb budget between forty-seven to fifty-three grams.

The Best Things to Eat at Pizza Hut: If you possess the willpower to only eat pizza toppings and leave the crust behind, your options at Pizza Hut widen substantially. Pick low-carb toppings like cheese, meats, and healthy veggies like peppers, onions, mushrooms, etc. Chicken wings are a low-carb winner here. Two pieces of mild wings contain less than one carb gram. You can eat two hot wings for the same single carb gram. Dip your wings in Blue Cheese dipping sauce for just two carbs. The ranch dipping sauce represents a lesser bargain at four grams. Best of all is lite ranch salad dressing, for zero carbs. You can accompany your wings or crustless pizza with a side order of green salad for about five or six net carbs. For dressing, choose lite ranch at zero carbs, Caesar at one gram, or ranch or Italian at two grams.

ROUND TABLE PIZZA
★★ | $–$$$

www.roundtablepizza.com

Over five hundred restaurants primarily in the western United States, with some international locations.

Claim to Fame: pizza

THE GOOD

If you have the willpower to eat the toppings off the pizza and leave the crust, your dining options widen. Choose your favorite combinations of meats, cheeses, and low-carb veggies. Otherwise salads and hot wings are the only truly low-carb choices here. Most Round Tables do offer salad bars, which makes it easy to build your own perfect low-carb salad with just the ingredients you like. By the time you read this, Round Table will have introduced a new reduced-carb pizza crust. Folks in the maintenance phase of a low-carb program will appreciate the thirty-percent fewer carbs, as compared to traditional pizza crust. Those on induction and weight-loss phases of the diet will still want to pass on the pizza crust. However, it's nice to know the option is there in case you ever need to minimize the damage a "falling-off-the-low-carb-wagon" pizza binge can bring.

THE BAD

Like all pizza restaurants, dough is the culprit here—pizza crusts and bread.

THE UGLY

A small three-piece order of garlic parmesan twists—Round Table's take on soft breadsticks—pack in seventy-one grams of carbs, fifty-nine grams for a piece of garlic cheese bread. Yow!

The Best Things to Eat at Round Table: A large order (six pieces) of buffalo wings contains only two carb grams. A large Caesar salad carries an effective carb count of nine net carbs. You can also have a large garden salad for twelve net carbs. Aside from that, order pizza or meat sandwiches and leave the bread or crust behind.

RYAN'S FAMILY STEAK HOUSE
★★★★★ | $–$$
www.ryans.com
Over 300 restaurants in twenty-three states.
Claim to Fame: reasonably priced steaks

THE GOOD

Steakhouses are always good low-carb choices, and this family favorite is no exception. You can build a custom low-carb meal by pairing your grilled steak (or chicken or salmon) with items from the Mega-Bar Buffet. Ryan's has also started implementing new low-carb menu items and plans to add more in the near future.

THE BAD

The same Mega-Bar Buffet that offers all those healthy low-carb choices also offers tons of illegal foods you'll have to resist.

THE UGLY

Some of the items on the Mega-Bar can do mega-damage to your weight loss plan. Steer far clear of pot pies, macaroni and cheese, spaghetti, cakes, cookies, pies, and other sweet or starchy items.

The Best Things to Eat at Ryan's Family Steakhouse: Order any of Ryan's steaks, sirloin tips, grilled chicken (without sauce), or grilled salmon for a virtually carb-free entrée. Some Ryan's restaurants also offer grilled pork chops, sausage, and other meat specials, and all contain less than four carbs per serving. In the evenings, you can always find freshly carved roast turkey, roast beef, and ham—all under two carbs per serving—at the Mega-Bar. Pair protein entrées with green salads and steamed or sautéed low-carb veggies like green beans, broccoli, cauliflower, sautéed mushrooms, collard greens, or cabbage, each under four net carbs. Finish your meal with a dish of sugar-free Jell-O topped with sugar-free whipped topping, for zero carbs. If your diet plan allows fruit, know that a 3.5-ounce serving of strawberries contains just five net carbs, seven for watermelon, or eight net carbs for cantaloupe. Want more desserts? A serving of sugar-free chocolate pudding weighs in at eleven net carbs, ten for sugar-free cookies.

SIZZLER RESTAURANT
★★★★★ | $$$

www.sizzler.com

Two hundred and forty restaurants across the western United States; limited restaurants in the northeast and midwest.

Claim to Fame: steaks

THE GOOD

From a low-carb standpoint, Sizzler is a great place to eat. The menu choices are staggering, from steaks, chicken, and seafood to an extensive salad bar. Almost all Sizzler Restaurants serve wine, so if your plan allows (or encourages) it, you can have a nice glass of vino with your dinner.

THE BAD

The salad bar at Sizzler is a great place to eat lots of healthy veggies, but be careful not to overload on higher-carb offerings. Skip the croutons, peas, and corn. Depending on the plan you're following and what stage of the diet you're on, beans and fruit may or may not be allowed—choose accordingly. Blue cheese, ranch, and vinegar and oil dressings are best. Dressings like Thousand Island or honey mustard contain too much sugar.

THE UGLY

Stay away from baked potatoes (which have a higher glycemic index than ice cream!), French fries, bread, or rice. Sizzler's salad bar comes with an appetizer and dessert bar. Stick to salad and don't go anywhere near the potato skins, pasta, batter-fried goodies, cakes, pies, and other desserts. If you can't control these urges, it's best to order off the menu and avoid the salad bar altogether.

The Best Things to Eat at Sizzler: Sizzler offers many great entrées, as long as you pass on potatoes or rice. Order steamed broccoli (about three net carbs) on the side instead. You can also add a side salad or a single trip to the salad bar to your entrée for a small extra fee. For about six net carbs, the sautéed mushrooms and grilled onions are a nice flavorful topping to any of Sizzler's no-carb steaks. Sizzlin' garlic herb chicken, Sizzlin' grilled shrimp skewers, or grilled salmon give diners plenty of non beef choices. Can't decide? Order a low-carb combo dinner: steak and lobster tail, steak and grilled shrimp skewers, or steak and shrimp scampi.

SOUPLANTATION/ SWEET TOMATOES
★★★★ | $$
www.sweettomatoes.com
Over ninety-five restaurants in fifteen states; concentrations in the west, southwest, midwest, and south.

Claim to Fame: all-you-can-eat soup, salad, pasta, and dessert bars

THE GOOD
There are tons of healthy high-fiber, low-carb foods to eat at these twin restaurants, which go by the moniker of Souplantation in California and Sweet Tomatoes in other areas of the country. You can custom-build your own salads with a huge array of low-carb ingredients such as spinach, field greens, romaine lettuce, cabbage, onions, peppers, tomatoes, cucumbers, bacon bits, cheese, cottage cheese, mushrooms, celery, cucumbers, sunflower seeds, and more, plus a host of prepared salads and nearly every variety of dressing imaginable. Low-carbers will also be able to indulge in many of Souplantation/Sweet Tomatoes' soups.

THE BAD
There's a dazzling display of muffins and breads up for grabs here. Don't indulge. A seemingly innocent maple walnut muffin carries an effective carb count of thirty-two grams; a piece of big-hearth pizza focaccia has fifteen.

THE UGLY
You'll find a huge assortment of desserts and sweet treats at these all-you-can-eat restaurants. At ten carb grams, you might be able to get away with a chocolate chip cookie, if you have the discipline to eat just one. Don't even think about the cobblers; a half-cup

serving of raspberry apple cobbler carries sixty-seven carb grams. You'll also want to avoid the carb-laden pasta bar entirely as a single cup serving will run you between twenty-eight to fifty-six grams, depending on sauce choices.

The Best Things to Eat at Souplantation/Sweet Tomatoes: (Portion sizes for soups and salads = one cup.) For the best low net-carb count salads choose the roasted vegetables with olives and feta, spinach gorgonzola with spiced pecans, California Cobb, or Cape Cod spinach with walnut or Greek salad (two net carbs). For just three net carbs, dish up a cup of Ensalada Azteca. For four net carbs try the classic Antipasto salad with peppered salami, Ranch house BLT salad with turkey, or the traditional spinach salad with bacon. For five effective carbs you can chow down on the country French salad with bacon, the vegetarian Indian summer spinach salad or the Mediterranean salad. The Roma tomato, mozzarella salad with basil will only cost you five net carbs.

You can also warm up with some hearty low-carb soups here. At just four carbs, your best bet by far is the low-fat chicken tortilla soup with jalapenos and tomatoes, followed by the Posole soup at six carbs and the vegetarian cream of broccoli soup and garlic kickin' roasted chicken soup at seven net carbs. For an effective carb count of eleven, try the broccoli onion soup, green chile stew, sweet tomato onion soup, vegetable medley soup, or vegetarian butternut squash soup. The Southwest tomato cream soup contains twelve net carbs. The broccoli cheese soup, cream of celery soup, old fashioned vegetable, and the Very Nice chicken and rice soup all have effective carb counts of thirteen grams.

Top off your Souplantation/Sweet Tomatoes meal with a dish of sugar-free Jell-O for zero carbs!

STEAK 'N SHAKE
★★★ | $
www.steakandshake.com

Over 400 restaurants in eighteen states, mostly in the south and midwest.

Claim to Fame: the "Steakburger" fries and shakes

THE GOOD

The quality of the meat here is so good, it's a real treat to order up a burger and eat it low-carb style—without the bun. Steak 'N Shake's Steakburgers are made from steak cuts of U.S. beef—sirloins, T-bones, and strip steaks—giving them fabulous flavor and juiciness. The Steak and Shake Web site has an innovative nutritional data calculator that figures the carb, fat, calorie (and more) counts for Steak and Shake food served just the way you like it. For instance, build a burger the way you like: no bread, add any combination of condiments like mustard, ketchup, mayonnaise, and add-ons like cheese, bacon, or mushrooms, and the nutrition calculator will let you know just how many carbs to budget for that meal. Low-carbers will also appreciate Steak and Shake's easy, inexpensive breakfast options.

THE BAD

Avoid the fries, onion rings, and bread on sandwiches; in other words, the usual high-carb suspects. A cup of chili at sixteen grams isn't the worst thing you could eat, but Steak and Shake offers better choices for the low-carb dieter. A 3.5-ounce serving of creamy cole slaw contains twenty-one carb grams. At nineteen carb grams, you'll also want to steer clear of the breaded fried fish filet. Cheating and leaving the bun on your burger will cost your daily carb budget twenty-nine grams. Even without the crisp tortilla shell, the taco salad contains 38.5 carb grams. Make that thirty-two grams for a shell-less chicken taco salad.

THE UGLY

Steak and Shake is part burger joint and part ice cream fountain, which means there's a lot of tempting sweet treats you'll need to resist. Stay away from the menu's extensive dessert section. Steak and Shake fries will also do major damage; a small order packs thirty-four grams of carbs, and at thirty-two carbs, a small order of onion rings isn't much better. Surprisingly, the worst carb offender is the old-fashioned baked beans, which contain seventy-six grams of carbohydrates. True, the beans also contain twelve grams of dietary fiber, but the resulting effective carb count remains an unacceptably high sixty-four grams.

The Best Things to Eat at Steak and Shake: Any of the Steakbugers, minus bread or bun, are great choices at Steak and Shake, as you can ask for just the condiments and accoutrements you prefer. The meat, cheese, and lettuce portions at Steak and Shake have zero carbs, as do fixings like mustard and mayonnaise. For just one carb gram, feel free to add two strips of bacon, and for two additional grams, you could top your Steakburger with sliced onion or tomato. A breadless turkey melt sandwich also provides a good carb bargain, as long as you eliminate the accompanying Frisco sauce, which is responsible for eleven of the dish's fourteen grams of carbohydrates. Seafood lovers can get five ounces of tuna salad for six carb grams. For side dishes, order the cottage cheese (without pineapple) for 3.5 grams or the small garden salad for four net carbs. You can also choose a main dish salad option—a chicken chef salad or deluxe garden salad have only 6.5 grams net carbs each.

Breakfast: Breakfasts are a breeze at Steak and Shake as the most popular no/low-carb morning favorites are all offered à la carte. For just a single gram of carbohydrates, you can have two eggs cooked in margarine, two slices of bacon, or a sausage patty. Those watching their cholesterol intake can order Healthy Morning cholesterol-free egg product (the equivalent of two eggs) prepared with margarine, for only two grams of carbs.

VILLAGE INN
★★★★ | $$
www.villageinnrestaurants.com
Over 200 restaurants with concentrations in the west, southwest, and midwest.
Claim to Fame: casual coffee-shop cuisine and pies

THE GOOD
Village Inn is one of the first coffee shops to jump onto the low-carb bandwagon. Their new carb-counter menu gives you lots of options for breakfast, lunch, and dinner—and keep in mind you can order breakfast items all day long.

THE BAD
Like most coffee shops, there are lots of high-carb foods to avoid here, but with so many low-carb choices, it's not hard to do.

THE UGLY
Some of the pies here look mighty tempting. Stay away from the dessert menu and save yourself forty or fifty or sixty carbs.

The Best Things to Eat at Village Inn: Village Inn's low-carb dinners, burgers, and melts all come accompanied with cottage cheese and a small dinner salad instead of the usual high-carb side dishes. Steamed veggies also come with the dinner. For about nine net carbs you can order a sirloin steak protein dinner or a grilled fish protein dinner. For about eleven net carbs, you can get two grilled center cut pork chops and the aforementioned sides. For about seventeen net carbs you can get the smothered grilled chicken protein dinner—two chicken breasts smothered with grilled peppers, onions, and mushrooms, and topped with Swiss cheese. The Ultimate Protein Double Burger consists of two, 1/3-pound burgers topped with bacon,

Swiss and American cheeses, lettuce, tomatoes, and pickles. The entire meal, including salad and cottage cheese, will cost you about nine net carb grams. The Protein Chicken Avocado Melt tops a grilled chicken breast with grilled onions, peppers, mushrooms, tomatoes, avocado, and melted cheese, for about thirteen carb grams. Salad lovers will appreciate the Protein Chef Salad at about eight net carb grams or the Protein Cobb Salad for about fifteen.

Breakfast: Village Inn doesn't forget low-carbers at breakfast either. No need to substitute or eliminate here; just order off the carb-counter menu, where most breakfasts come with cottage cheese instead of the usual bread and potatoes. For under four carb grams, choose any of the classic egg combos: sausage, bacon, ham, steak, ground beef patty, or pork chops, and eggs. For about three grams each, you can also order the Three-Meat Protein Omelet or the Ham and Cheese Protein Omelet. The Southwestern Chicken Protein Omelet and the Denver Protein Omelet modestly weigh in at about five grams each.

WAFFLE HOUSE
★★★★ | $–$$
www.wafflehouse.com

Over 1,400 restaurants in twenty-five states, with concentrations in the south and midwest.

Claim to Fame: waffles, breakfast items, casual diner-type food

THE GOOD

You can get a large variety of no- and low-carb foods at Waffle House, twenty-four hours a day, seven days a week.

"Low carb is nothing new to us," says Waffle House communications director Pat Warner. "We've been around so long, we've seen this trend before and we're now experiencing the resurgence. We've always been a cook-to-order restaurant, so people can get just what they want."

THE BAD

Skip the fries, onion rings, and bread on burgers and sandwiches.

THE UGLY

While they're known for them, the waffles at Waffle House will break the carb bank to the tune of thirty diet-busting carb grams or more.

The Best Things to Eat at Waffle House: You'll find lots of no- and ultra-low-carb entrées served à la carte or in combinations at Waffle House—steaks, chopped steaks, pork chops, ham, and grilled chicken, not to mention breakfast—twenty-four hours a day—with eggs, bacon, sausage, and omelets. Order sliced tomatoes (about four net carbs) or a small garden salad (about three net carbs) to go with your meals instead of the usual high-starch sides. Waffle House also offers a decent selection of low-carb entrée-sized salads, none which should run over ten net carbs (without croutons and dressing): BLT salad, chef's salad, and grilled chicken or ribeye steak salads.

WESTERN SIZZLIN'
★★★★★ | $–$$
www.westernsizzlin.com
Over 150 restaurants in twenty-two states.
Claim to Fame: steaks

THE GOOD
Western Sizzlin' offers lots of protein entrées, low-carb salads and side dishes, and even sugar-free gelatin for dessert.

THE BAD
This restaurant's all-you-can-eat buffet also offers lots of high-carb items.

THE UGLY
In addition, the buffet also offers some offensively high-carb items like pies and cakes and other desserts.

The Best Things to Eat at Western Sizzlin': Choose your favorite cut of steak for zero carbs. Pair it with some low-carb steamed veggies and build your perfect low-carb salad at the salad bar. If you don't feel like a steak, you can also get roasted chicken, broiled or grilled fish, roast turkey, pork loin, or roast beef. Finish your meal with a bowl of zero carb, sugar-free Jell-O.

Breakfast: Some Western Sizzlin' locations offer all-you-can-eat breakfast buffets every day, some on weekends, some not at all. Check with your restaurant as it's a great low-carb way to start the day. Pick and choose just the foods you want: eggs, bacon, ham, sausage—even oatmeal and other cereals.

Midrange Restaurants

APPLEBEE'S NEIGHBORHOOD GRILL & BAR
★★★ | $$–$$$$
www.applebees.com
Over 1,500 restaurants in forty-nine states and nine countries.
Claim to Fame: American food

THE GOOD
Low-carbers can always find lots of choices at Applebee's, including steaks, chicken, seafood, and salads. Menu offerings change by region, so you might even find more choices than those listed below.

THE BAD
Avoid most appetizers. Aside from buffalo wings, they all contain bread in some form. Beware—there's lots of sugar in the sauces that come on many of Applebee's entrées. Avoid anything with honey or barbecue in the title or item description, or ask for no sauce.

THE UGLY
Triple Chocolate Meltdown Cake. Need I say more? Don't even look at Applebee's dessert menu. There are also lots of tempting sweet drinks to order from the bar. Stick to red wine, light beer, or no-carb alcohols like rum, vodka, or gin with sugar-free mixers, if you must drink at all.

The Best Things to Eat at Applebee's: Start your meal with an order of buffalo chicken wings (less than one gram of carbs) with blue cheese dressing and celery sticks.

At zero carbs, you can't do any better than the steaks. Order them with a green salad and steamed veggies and you've got a great low-carb meal. You can get grilled chicken or salmon as well, but make sure to tell your server no honey glaze or barbecue sauce, as these can add ten or more carb grams. The grilled chicken Caesar or Santa Fe chicken salads are great choices, too, but to keep the carbs under eight grams, ask the kitchen to hold the croutons or tortilla strips.

BAHAMA BREEZE
★★★★ | $$$$–$$$$$

www.bahamabreeze.com

Over forty restaurants in twenty-one states.

Claim to Fame: Caribbean cuisine

THE GOOD
The Caribbean-inspired cuisine at this casual eatery provides a nice change to the typical flavors found at most chain restaurants. For low-carbers, there are steaks, pork, chicken, and seafood, all served with an island flair.

THE BAD
Stay away from the wood-fired pizzas, pastas, and sandwiches. Be careful with salads, too; many of them here have sweet dressings like tropical vinaigrette or high-carb ingredients such as sweet corn or tamarind-glazed tomatoes that make them undesirable.

THE UGLY
Forget about desserts, especially the Pina Colada bread pudding. Can a dessert get more carb-laden than bread pudding?

The Best Things to Eat at Bahama Breeze: Start your meal with an order of Habenero Wings (Bahama Breeze's version of buffalo wings). For entrées try the oak-grilled filet mignon or New York strip steaks (zero carbs); pan-seared pork tenderloins (zero carbs without the rum demiglace sauce); ancho-rubbed grilled chicken breast (about two carbs); jumbo sea scallops with chimichurri or seared ahi tuna with wasabi cream sauce (about four grams). For side dishes, order some steamed veggies (about four net carbs) and a small Caesar salad (about three net carbs without croutons) or garden salad (about six net carbs). For about eight net carbs, the sun-ripened Tomato salad—a mixture of red grape, yellow pear, and beefsteak tomatoes—gives low-carbers something a little out of the ordinary. Skip the tropical or citrus vinaigrette dressings that normally come on these salads and use carb-free vinegar and oil instead.

BENNIGAN'S GRILL & TAVERN
★★★ | $$–$$$$

www.bennigans.com

Over 300 restaurants throughout the United States as well as some international locations.

Claim to Fame: Irish-American pub fare

THE GOOD
Bennigan's has a new low-carb menu, making it easy to order directly off the menu without substitutions and special requests. You'll also find some terrific creative salads.

THE BAD
Appetizers at Bennigan's are off-limits, including the usually low-carb buffalo wings; Bennigan's are breaded.

THE UGLY
Bennigan's offers some truly decadent frozen drinks that are way off the carb scale, along with lots of tempting desserts. Death by Chocolate says it all—stay away!

The Best Things to Eat at Bennigan's: For about ten carb grams, you can start your meal with a cup of chicken noodle soup. You can never go wrong with steak, and Bennigan's has a wide variety to choose from. The O'Cajun Salmon gives you a flaky, grilled, seven-ounce filet seasoned with spicy Cajun seasonings, for nine carb grams. You can also get two seasoned thick grilled pork chops (ten grams). Keep in mind the carbs in these dishes primarily come from the low-carb vegetable sides, green beans or steamed broccoli. Bennigan's also offers some low-carb bunless sandwiches: the American burger (ten grams), the Big Irish burger (eleven grams) and the bacon & cheese burger (nine grams). The grilled chicken or grilled salmon Caesar salads are great bets, at about ten grams, providing you leave off the croutons. Bennigan's club salad also fits the bill with a mixture of turkey, cheeses, cucumber, bacon, and tomatoes. The ahi tuna steak salad is a welcome change to the usual chicken, but be sure to ask your server to leave off the fried wontons and choose a no-carb vinegar and oil dressing instead of the sweet sesame ginger vinaigrette that typically comes with it.

BIG BOWL ASIAN KITCHEN
★★★ | $$–$$$
www.bigbowl.com
Twenty restaurants in seven states: Colorado, Illinois, Minnesota, North Carolina, Texas, Virginia, and Wisconsin.
Claim to Fame: Asian cuisine

THE GOOD
Big Bowl's Stir-Fry Bar—you may know it as Mongolian barbecue—allows diners to pick and choose their own vegetables in the ratios they like, then add seasonings and sauces and their choice of protein. The dish is then quickly stir-fried to perfection.

THE BAD
This is an Asian restaurant; everything comes with rice or noodles of some sort.

THE UGLY
Some of the dishes on the menu, like crispy orange peel shrimp or chicken, are battered, fried, and then coated with sweet sauces or glazes. Anything with teriyaki or sweet and sour sauce will also have tons of sugar.

The Best Things to Eat at Big Bowl Asian Kitchen: There's really only one choice here, but it's a good one—the Stir-Fry Bar. Start by filling your bowl with your favorite low-carb vegetables. Then choose beef, chicken, shrimp, salmon, or tofu. Next choose a sauce; low-carbers should choose the Chinese Ginger Garlic Sauce or the Vegetarian Mushroom Sauce. Skip the noodles or rice that usually accompany this meal. The carb count will depend on which ingredients and the amount of ingredients you choose. Stick to legal, low-carb veggies and no-carb meats. The sauces shouldn't add more than a handful of grams.

BUCA DI BEPPO
★★★★ | $$–$$$$
www.bucadibeppo.com
Over ninety restaurants in thirty states.
Claim to Fame: southern Italian cuisine

THE GOOD
You'll be pleased to find a surprisingly large number of low-carb menu choices—even pasta—at these festive Italian restaurants where all dishes are served family style and meant for sharing. Gather your low-carbing friends and have a feast—Buca di Beppo specializes in parties for groups as small as two and as large as one hundred. You can even reserve a table right in the kitchen!

THE BAD
This is an Italian restaurant; you'll need to resist the pasta and the fabulous bread. The portions here are huge, even the small dishes. Don't be a member of the clean plate club; share your dishes among your party and don't be afraid to take some home.

THE UGLY
Buca di Beppo serves some great desserts, including a family-sized portion of tiramisu. Luckily, you'll probably be so full from the meal, you won't be able to indulge, even if your willpower is slipping.

The Best Things to Eat at Buca di Beppo: Since all dishes at Buca di Beppo are served family-style and meant to be shared, the net carb counts below are based upon a 3.5-ounce (100-gram) serving and rounded to the closest carb.

Start your meal with the cold antipasti platter at three net carbs per serving or some fresh mozzarella caprese for seven. Seafood lovers should order the mussels marinara at four grams or the fried calamari at eight.

Here's a worthwhile secret; special for carb-counters but not listed on the Buca menu is the Latini Meat Platter with Vesuvio Tomatoes. Ask your server about this special combo dish of roasted chicken, pork chops, beef tenderloin, and sausage (hot or mild), served with stuffed tomatoes. The meat portion of the Latini Meat Platter contains less than one carb gram, the Vesuvio tomatoes weigh in at six grams per serving. Other low-carb entrées include the chicken with lemon or the chicken Saltimbocca, for two net carbs per serving; the shrimp parmagiana for three or the shrimp scampi for four. Pasta lovers can indulge their cravings with baked cannelloni for five net carbs per serving or baked manicotti for nine net carbs. For side dishes, order the Di Beppo salad or the mixed green salad with prosciutto and gorgonzola for two net carbs each or the Caesar salad for six net carbs per serving. Eat your veggies by ordering escarole for two net carbs or green beans for three. Buca also offers side orders of sausage (one carb per serving) and meatballs (four net carbs).

CALIFORNIA PIZZA KITCHEN
★★ | $$–$$$
www.cpk.com
Found in twenty-eight states and parts of Asia.
Claim to Fame: California-style pizza

THE GOOD
Salads rule at CPK. They also serve espresso and cappuccino, so you can relax and have something to sip while other diners have dessert.

THE BAD
Skip the usual suspects—bread, pasta, rice, potatoes, and desserts. None of the regular menu appetizers at California Pizza Kitchen are going to do your low-carb diet any good, either. The hummus would be fine on some plans (such as the South Beach Diet), but the bread they serve to dip it in is off-limits (unless you're on maintenance).

THE UGLY
Pizza is tough to resist for many people, so if the aroma of freshly baking dough is going to break your willpower, find a different restaurant. My niece, who lost over a hundred pounds on a low-carb diet and has kept it off for over two years now, regularly goes to pizza restaurants and eats just the toppings. I don't have that kind of willpower, but if you do, your menu options at CPK increase dramatically.

The Best Things to Eat at California Pizza Kitchen: CPK's Original Chopped Salad, with lettuce, basil, salami, roast turkey breast, tomatoes, scallions, and cheese tossed with herb-mustard parmesan vinaigrette, runs about six net carbs. Order the smoked bacon and gorgonzola salad, but ask your server to leave off the buttermilk batter-fried onions that usually top this salad of chopped lettuce, basil, applewood-smoked bacon, Gorgonzola cheese, jicama, red cabbage, and diced tomatoes (about eleven net carbs). The white balsamic salad Provençal—greens, arugula, red cabbage, feta cheese, sun-dried tomatoes, Mediterranean olives, and Roma tomatoes with a white balsamic vinaigrette—contains about thirteen net carbs. You can also order a classic Caesar or chicken Caesar salad. If you skip the croutons, you'll bring the effective carb count down to about five to six grams.

CHEESECAKE FACTORY
★★★★★ | $$–$$$
www.cheesecakefactory.com
Over seventy-five restaurants in twenty-five states.
Claim to Fame: bistro fare, cheesecakes

THE GOOD
Cheesecake Factory's enormous menu offers low-carbers lots of choices from creative salads and meat entrées to vegetable side dishes. You can also get omelets all day long. While it's not perfected as of this writing, Cheesecake Factory sources tell me a low-carb cheesecake is in the works. Oh, happy day!

THE BAD
Lurking within that huge menu are lots of high-carb items: breaded fried appetizers, quesadillas, sandwiches, potatoes, pizza, pastas, and more.

THE UGLY
With a name like the Cheesecake Factory, do I really need to tell you what to avoid here?

The Best Things to Eat at Cheesecake Factory: Cheesecake Factory prides itself on accommodating customer's dietary needs, so don't be afraid to mix and match side dishes with entrées to get what you need. You'll find more choices than most restaurants, including steamed asparagus and broccoli (about three net carbs each) along with sautéed snow peas and mixed vegetables (about seven net carbs) and spinach (about four grams). Entrée choices are myriad. Try lemon-herb roasted chicken, crusted chicken romano (chicken coated in a delicious romano and parmesan cheese crust), herb-crusted filet of salmon, blackened shrimp New Orleans, marinated grilled pork chops, grilled skirt steak, cajun ribeye steak, or filet mignon. Check for daily seafood specials as well. Many of these entrées are carbless; none will have more than a handful of grams. You can also get an order of buffalo wings (less than half a gram per wing) as a starter or main course. Omelets are another great choice at Cheesecake Factory. Create your own low- or no-carb omelet with favorite ingredients like bacon, ham, cheese, mushrooms, spinach, pepper, and onions. In addition, the menu offers several tasty omelet combinations: Joe's Special (chicken sausage, spinach, mushrooms, and onions, about six net carbs); California omelet (avocado, mushrooms, green onion, tomato, sour cream, three cheeses, and a touch of garlic and shallots, about eleven net carbs); Rustic Garden omelet (grilled eggplant, zucchini, asparagus, peppers, tomato, red onion, and melted cheese) or the asparagus, portobello, and artichoke omelet (also includes cheese and tomatoes, with about 15 net carbs each.

Cheesecake Factory also offers some wonderful salads (lunch-sized portions of most salads available until five P.M.). Try the Caesar or chicken Caesar (without croutons) or the herb-crusted salmon salad for about six net carbs each, or the Cobb salad for about eight to ten net carbs each. For more variety, fiber, and nutrients order the Symphony Salad—a combination of grilled chicken, tomatoes, asparagus, red and yellow peppers, green beans, fresh mozzarella, and butter lettuce with parmesan cheese, for about twelve net carbs.

CHEVYS
★★★ | $–$$
www.chevys.com
Over 120 restaurants in sixteen states, with concentrations in the west.
Claim to Fame: fresh Mexican cuisine

THE GOOD
Chevys offers some great salad choices with interesting dressings. The fajitas are fairly low in carbs, too.

THE BAD
Most menu choices here come on or in some sort of tortilla, which means refined carbs. Eat the fillings, not the wrappings, and you can keep the carb count low at Chevys.

THE UGLY
Chevys offers some carb-laden desserts including traditional flan, caramel empanadas, and ice cream sundaes—steer clear.

The Best Things to Eat at Chevys: A serving of chicken, steak, fish, or shrimp fajitas will only run you about thirteen carbs; sixteen for veggie fajitas or broiled or grilled fish with San Antonio vegetables (onions and peppers with spices) and salsa, but without tortillas. Cut more carbs by asking your server to leave the potatoes off the grilled veggies, which also include squash, broccoli, carrots, and asparagus. A half-cup of black or refried beans has an effective carb count of about thirteen grams.

Ask your server to leave the roasted corn salsa off the Santa Fe chopped salad for a low-carb meal that combines romaine lettuce, avocado, mesquite grilled chicken, bacon, and crumbled blue cheese, for about nine net carbs. The Tostada salad is another good bargain, providing you don't eat the fried tortilla shell (have or skip the refried beans as your particular diet plan permits). Chevys makes a unique chicken Caesar salad as well, with mesquite-grilled chicken, fire-roasted peppers, and Mexican Cotijo cheese, for about eight net carbs. Top your salads with one of Chevys great low-carb dressing choices: classic Caesar, creamy ranch, Chipotle Aioli, or salsa vinaigrette. None of the dressings should cost over four grams per tablespoon.

CHI-CHI'S
★★★ | $$–$$$

www.chi-chis.com
Over sixty restaurants in thirteen states, mostly
East Coast and midwest.
Claim to Fame: Mexican cuisine

THE GOOD
Salads and grilled entrées give low-carbers more
choices than many other Mexican restaurants.

THE BAD
All of Chi-Chi's appetizers are high-carb and off
limits. All menu items come on or in tortillas, which
you'll need to resist. When ordering salads, ask your
server to leave the fried tortilla bowl in the kitchen
and serve your salad on a plate instead.

THE UGLY
Chi-Chi's offers two truly disastrously high-carb desserts: Mexican deep-fried ice cream and Chocolate
Meltdown Cake. Need I tell you that either of these
will stop weight loss progress in its tracks?

The Best Things to Eat at Chi Chi's: The taco salad
combines your choice of seasoned ground beef, shredded
beef, grilled steak, grilled or blackened chicken, or seafood
on a bed of lettuce topped with shredded cheese, fresh
tomatoes, and sour cream, for about ten to twelve net
carbs. You can also order the Ensalada de la Casa, a tasty
melange of lettuce, cabbage, carrots, pico de gallo, and
shredded cheese, for about four net carbs.

Chi-Chi's has some terrific low-carb grilled entrées
including a flat iron steak (zero carbs), fire-grilled shrimp
skewers (fourteen carbs), and fire-grilled citrus and herb
marinated chicken breasts (eight carbs). For side dishes,
skip the rice, mashed potatoes, or corn cakes, and order

an Ensalada de la Casa or an order of steamed or sautéed southwest vegetables—a medley of zucchini, squash, onions, and peppers. If your diet plan allows beans, an order of Chi-Chi's pinto beans have an effective carb count of about nineteen grams.

CHILI'S
★★★ | $–$$$

www.chilis.com
Over 900 restaurants in forty-nine states and twenty-three countries.
Claim to Fame: southwest and Mexican cuisine

THE GOOD
While Chili's has always prepared food to order and accommodated customers' special requests and substitutions, their new "It's Your Choice" menu makes ordering low-carb meals easy.

THE BAD
This is a Southwest/Mexican restaurant so there are lots of tortilla-wrapped foods.

THE UGLY
The Awesome Blossom is a huge sweet onion, coated with high-carb batter and deep fried—awesomely high in carbs. Avoid Chili's extensive dessert menu, too.

The Best Things to Eat at Chili's: Begin your meal with a pound of spicy unbreaded chicken wings served with blue cheese dressing for nearly no carbs. For zero carbs order a flame-grilled ribeye steak. The Monterey chicken (grilled chicken breast with applewood smoked bacon, cheese, and tomatoes) weighs in at about four to six carbs, providing you skip the BBQ sauce that normally comes with it. Chili's fajita Caesar salad includes marinated beef or chicken on romaine lettuce with Caesar dressing and topped with parmesan cheese, for about ten net carbs. You'll find three bunless low-carb burgers, all served with steamed vegetables: the Oldtimer (with lettuce, tomato, onion, and pickles), Bacon Burger, or Mushroom-Swiss Burger, for a mere handful of carbs each. You can also ask for "Knife and

Fork" chicken or beef fajitas served over fresh vegetables with pico de gallo, cheese, guacamole, and sour cream, for about ten to twelve net carbs.

COZYMEL'S COASTAL MEXICAN GRILL
★★★ | $$–$$$

www.cozymels.com

Fifteen restaurants in ten states: Arkansas, California, Georgia, Illinois, Kansas, Nevada, New York, Ohio, Tennessee, and Texas.

Claim to Fame: coastal Mexican grill

THE GOOD
Cozymel's offers lettuce-wrapped fajitas, so low-carbers can chow down without tortilla-associated guilt.

THE BAD
Like most Mexican restaurants, many menu items at Cozymel's come in or on tortillas and are accompanied by rice and/or beans, so order with caution or be prepared to leave food on your plate.

THE UGLY
You don't even have to belly up to the bar at Cozymel's to be tempted by exotic sweet cocktails and margaritas. There are also some decadent desserts that you'll need to ignore.

The Best Things to Eat at Cozymel's: Lettuce-wrapped fajitas rule at Cozymel's, and you can get a huge variety of them—steak, chicken, pork, shrimp, ahi tuna, and portobello mushrooms and veggies. The meat should be zero carbs; you can eat about six lettuce leaves for less than two net carbs; a cup of the mushrooms and veggies should run in the eight to ten net carb range. You can also get entrée-sized Caesar salads, with or without chicken, shrimp, or salmon. If you skip the crispy tortilla puffs that usually add crunch to these salads, they should run about six to eight net carbs.

You can also order several low-carb entrées, providing you substitute a small salad and steamed or sautéed veggies for the usual rice, beans, and tortillas. Many of these entrées come with Cozymel's salsas or cream sauces. None should cost you more five or so grams of carbs, depending on how much sauce you consume. Use this handy tip to get just a taste of the sauces you love without adding unnecessary carbs: dip the tines of your fork in the sauce, then use the fork to pick up the food. You'll get the essence of the taste you crave without all the accompanying carbs. The meat portion of the following entrées weigh in between zero and four carbs (how much the meal totals will depend on the amount of sides and sauces you consume); the Shrimp Mojo de Ajo (pan-seared shrimp, seasonal vegetables, and roasted garlic tossed in a light vino blanco); Carne Asada (marinated Mexican steak, flame-grilled and topped with ranchero sauce); Pork Rotistado (slow-roasted pork with seasonal vegetables); or Pollo Poblano (grilled chicken topped with poblano cream sauce and seasonal vegetables).

DAVE & BUSTER'S
★★★ | $$–$$$

www.daveandbusters.com

Over thirty restaurants in fourteen states: California, Colorado, Florida, Georgia, Hawaii, Illinois, Maryland, Michigan, Missouri, New York, Ohio, Pennsylvania, Rhode Island, and Texas, plus Toronto, Mexico City, and Taipei.

Claim to Fame: American food in an atmosphere of fun and games

THE GOOD

Steaks, grilled salmon, and a salad or two give low-carbers a variety of food choices here. Even though Dave & Buster's offers lots of tempting high-carb items on their menu, their extensive variety of high-tech games and amusements provide great diversions from thoughts of deprivation.

THE BAD

All the appetizers are off-limits, even the usually low-carb buffalo wings, as Dave & Buster's breads theirs. Most salads here contain high-carb ingredients or sweet dressings, so order carefully.

THE UGLY

Avoid all desserts and sweet drinks.

The Best Things to Eat at Dave & Buster's: Dave & Buster's recently introduced new low-carb menu items including the Double Cheeseburger Stack (zero carbs for cheese and meat; add in your desired toppings and condiments); gorgonzola sirloin or ribeye steaks and peppered steaks (zero carbs); chargrilled salmon and green beans (about five net carbs); grilled chicken Caesar salad (without croutons); and chicken Monte Carlo, made up of lemon herb chicken, Boursin cheese, and red peppers (about six net carbs each); and the BLT salad (eleven net carbs). For side dishes, choose sautéed mushrooms (about two net carbs), green beans (about 3.5), or a small green salad (about three net carbs).

DON PABLO'S
★★★ | $$–$$$
www.donpablos.com
Over a hundred restaurants in nineteen eastern states.
Claim to Fame: Mexican cuisine

THE GOOD
Don Pablo's was one of the first major chains to jump on the low-carb bandwagon. Not only do they offer low-carb foods like lettuce-wrapped fajitas, they even have a low-carb margarita!

THE BAD
As this is Mexican food, beware of anything in a tortilla, aside from the low-carb menu. Most of the entrée salads also have high-carb ingredients; even the Caesar salad comes with honey-roasted pecans and tortilla strips.

THE UGLY
Don's has some great desserts that low-carbers can't eat, including classic Mexican sopapillas—fried puff pastries covered in powdered sugar. It doesn't get much worse than that.

The Best Things to Eat at Don Pablo's: Fajitas—Don Pablo's serves them on a bed of grilled, fire-roasted low-carb veggies: yellow squash, zucchini, mushrooms, and asparagus. Instead of the traditional tortilla, wrap your fajitas in crisp iceberg lettuce. The mesquite-grilled Black Angus steak or sautéed mahi-mahi fajitas weigh in at fifteen net carbs each; the grilled smoked chicken variety contains about eighteen net carbs. The vegetables in these menu options account for about eight net carbs, with three coming from Don Pablo's special sauce. Your can add four grilled jumbo shrimp (zero carbs) to any entrée for a small additional charge. For only 1.5 carb grams, accompany your meal with a hand-shaken or frozen low-carb margarita made from fresh-squeezed lime juice, low-carb margarita mix, and a shot of gold tequila.

EL CHICO
★★★ | $$–$$$

www.elchico.com
Nearly a hundred restaurants in the south and southwest.

Claim to Fame: Mexican cuisine

THE GOOD
If you look closely, you'll find some good low-carb grilled entrées and salads on El Chico's menu.

THE BAD
There are lots of high-carb items and tortilla-wrapped foods to avoid here, as well as the typical Mexican side dishes, rice and beans.

THE UGLY
Forget about desserts, especially, but not limited to, the sopapillas (fried pastries) filled with honey and dusted with cinnamon sugar, deep-fried ice cream, or brownie skillet sundae.

The Best Things to Eat at El Chico: Try the chicken fajita salad (grilled chicken, cheddar cheese, tomatoes, and guacamole over salad greens) for about eleven net carbs. From El Chico's grill order the ribeye steak (zero carbs) or the chicken Monterey (grilled chicken breast topped with grilled onions, mushrooms, and peppers, and topped with melted Jack cheese), for about eight net carbs each. You can also order a plain grilled chicken breast or bunless double cheeseburger from El Chico's American menu. For side dishes, order sautéed vegetables or a small green salad, for between three and six net carbs.

FAMOUS DAVE'S LEGENDARY PIT BAR-B-QUE
★★★ | $$–$$$
www.famousdaves.com
Over ninety restaurants in twenty-three states.
Claim to Fame: award-winning barbecue

THE GOOD
There are lots of meats to be had at Famous Dave's—always good news for low-carbers. As I write this, Famous Dave's is test marketing some new low-carb plates. Keep checking their Web site for new developments.

THE BAD
While most of Dave's meats are carb-legal, his barbecue sauces are not. If your protein of choice can't be served without the delicious but off-limit sauce, don't order it. This is down-home comfort food at its finest. Likewise, a lot of menu items will be off limits including drunken apples, cornbread muffins, and cole slaw. Dave's double smoked ham is cooked and basted in a sweet glaze, so avoid this protein option.

THE UGLY
They cook up some fabulous down-home desserts at Famous Dave's. Of course, low-carbers can't indulge in such things as Dave's Famous Bread Pudding, Better Than Mom's Pecan Pie, or hot fudge Kahlua brownies.

The Best Things to Eat at Famous Dave's: Baby back pork or beef ribs, pulled pork, or beef brisket can all be served without barbecue sauce, giving them carb counts of near zero. In the same zero to one carb range is the country roasted lemon pepper chicken, the buffalo chicken wings, and the hot links sausages. Unfortunately, low-carb side dish options are limited to a small Caesar salad (about four net carbs without croutons) or garden salad (about six net carbs). For about eight to ten net carbs (without croutons), you can also get a meal-sized Caesar salad, with or without grilled chicken.

HARD ROCK CAFÉ
★★★ | $$–$$$$

www.hardrockcafe.com

Over a hundred restaurants in the metropolitan areas of forty-four countries.

Claim to Fame: burgers and casual food in a rock and roll atmosphere

THE GOOD

Salads, steaks, and chicken will give low-carbers enough menu choices to indulge in while their omnivorous friends chow down on burgers and fries. HRC also serves Rolling Rock Green Light beer.

THE BAD

Hard Rock Café offers many "really big" sandwiches and burgers that come on bread, accompanied by French fries. You'll also want to avoid Hard Rock's "Smokehouse" menu, as the items all come slathered in high-carb BBQ sauce.

THE UGLY

Hard Rock has a huge dessert menu filled with enough carbs to blow the diets of a small midwestern town. As if regular appetizer nachos aren't bad enough, HRC makes dessert nachos! The restaurant even has their own signature ice cream that's integral to many of the off-limits desserts. The drinks menu is overflowing with creative, sweet cocktails. If you must drink, stick to light beer, wine, or carb-free drinks like rum and diet cola.

The Best Things to Eat at Hard Rock Café: Like many casual American restaurants, you can get virtually carb-free buffalo wings served with celery and blue cheese dressing at the Hard Rock. For entrées, order the Texas T-bone steak, herb-marinated chicken breast or the grilled catch of the day. Specify no sauces and your entrée should have zero carbs. You can substitute a small garden or Caesar salad (about four to six net carbs without croutons) and sautéed vegetables for the usual starchy high-carb side dishes. HRC also offers entrée-sized Caesar salads (about nine net carbs) and Cobb salads (about fifteen net carbs) as well as a mixed vegetable house salad that you can enhance with your favorite no-carb ingredients like grilled chicken, smoked turkey breast, shrimp, bacon, egg, and cheese. Wash it all down with a bottle of Rolling Rock's Rock Green Light low-carb beer.

HOOTER'S
★★★★ | $$–$$$

www.hooters.com
Over 300 restaurants in forty-four states and thirteen countries.
Claim to Fame: casual food served by gorgeous women

THE GOOD
Lots of steamed seafood options give low-carb dieters something a little out of the ordinary at Hooters.

THE BAD
A big part of Hooter's menu is sandwiches; luckily there are enough other items to not make them a temptation.

THE UGLY
Stay away from the curly fries, jalapeno chili cheese fries, macaroni salad, potato salad, and desserts.

The Best Things to Eat at Hooter's: You can pig out on ten of Hooter's naked (unbreaded) buffalo chicken wings for less than a single carb gram. You'll also find a dizzying array of steamed seafood all carb-free: raw or steamed oysters on the half shell, Carolina-style roast oysters, steamed snow crab legs, peel-and-eat shrimp, or steamed clams. Want something a little different? Try Hooter's Smoysters Rockefeller—steamed oysters on the half shell smothered in bacon and provolone cheese. If you order the Hooter's Shooter (oyster cocktail), you even get to take home the collector's shot glass it comes in.

Hooter's also offer some decent low-carb salads. Lowest in carbs (about eight net carbs without croutons or tortilla strips) are the grilled chicken Caesar or the Southwest fiesta salad. For about twelve net carbs, try the grilled chicken garden salad (again, pass on the croutons).

HOULIHAN'S
★★★★★ | $$–$$$$

www.houlihans.com
Over eighty restaurants across the United States
and in Puerto Rico and Mexico.
Claim to Fame: casual American food

THE GOOD
If a new low-carb menu plus lots of low-carb items on
the regular menu wasn't enough to get you to go to
Houlihan's, think about their Skinny Mini Chocolate
Mousse dessert for just four net carbs.

THE BAD
Forget about starchy sides and appetizers—and there
are some tempting ones here—Houlihan's even
makes their own potato chips. There are also a lot of
breaded and fried entrées and appetizers.

THE UGLY
Desserts, as always, are the dieter's downfall, including a Chocolate Candy Sundae—four (count them)
scoops of ice cream with crushed Snickers and Reese's
Peanut Butter Cups, drizzled with hot fudge and caramel. It doesn't get much sweeter than that, folks.

The Best Things to Eat at Houlihan's: Order some
buffalo wings as an appetizer or entrée—you can have
four wings for less than a single carb gram. For meal-sized
salads, try the classic Caesar salad with or without grilled
chicken or salmon for about six net carbs, providing you
skip the croutons.

All of Houlihan's entrées come with fresh broccoli and
their innovative California Mashers, both of which are
reflected in the carb counts that follow. This delicious
mashed potato stand-in is made from mashed cauliflower,
real butter, cream cheese, and roasted garlic, and can be

topped with melted cheese or bacon. Cauliflower has always been a great diet bargain, but prepared this way, it's also a great taste sensation.

For 5.4 net carbs you can get a low-carb burger and for a couple of extra grams, you can augment it with optional toppings like sautéed mushrooms, bacon, cheese, or blue cheese. At 5.6 net carbs, enjoy the prime top sirloin dinner; for 6.1 net carbs, you can pair a top sirloin steak with a skewer of four jumbo grilled shrimp. The low-carb coriander grilled salmon dinner will cost your daily budget 6.4 net carbs; seven for the grilled shrimp. Finally, 7.2 grams buys you a double grilled rosemary chicken breast, basted in red wine and garlic butter.

Best of all you can finish your meal with dessert—Houlihan's Skinny Mini Chocolate Mousse, for just four net carb grams.

LONE STAR STEAKHOUSE & SALOON
★★★★★ | $$$–$$$$

www.lonestarsteakhouse.com
Two hundred and fifty restaurants, with concentrations in the east.
Claim to Fame: steaks

THE GOOD
Great steaks, grilled chicken and fish, ribs, and even pork chops, served with a nice variety of sides and salads—what more could a low-carb dieter want?

THE BAD
The desserts here are bad, but luckily it's a very limited menu.

THE UGLY
The worst things to eat here are the baked potato, at 111 net carbs and the baked sweet potato, at 137 grams.

The Best Things to Eat at Lone Star Steakhouse & Saloon: Take your choice of a wide range of no-carb protein entrées including eight different mesquite-grilled steaks, prime rib, grilled chicken, pork chops, Sweet Bourbon Salmon, and ribs. Some of these entrées come with BBQ, honey mustard, or other sweet sauces, but just ask your server to leave them off in order to keep the carb count at zero. You can also order grilled shrimp for less than two carbs. Pair your entrée with a side salad (about five net carbs without croutons), steamed vegetables (about six), sautéed mushrooms (one net carb) or sautéed onions (seven). You can also enjoy a cup of Lone Star Chili for about seven net carbs. The El Paso garden salad has an effective carb count of about nine, providing you skip the croutons. The chicken Caesar salad (again without croutons) will run you about six net carbs.

LONGHORN STEAKHOUSE
★★★★★ | $$$ - $$$$

www.longhornsteakhouse.com
Nearly 200 restaurants in twenty-three eastern and midwest states.
Claim to Fame: steaks

THE GOOD
Not only does this western-style steakhouse offer a wide variety of protein entrées, above and beyond great steaks, they have a respectable number of low-carb sides as well.

THE BAD
Forget about the baked or sweet potatoes, which can easily run forty or more grams of carbs.

THE UGLY
Desserts are the culprit here, including (would you believe?) a breaded fried cheesecake. Can you feel your arteries clogging?

The Best Things to Eat at LongHorn SteakHouse: Of course, the steaks are terrific and there's a large selection to choose from. For a different low-carb take on steak, try Longhorn's Bleu Cheese Crusted Filet—a nine-ounce filet, cooked to order, and topped with melted bleu cheese, served over a marinated, grilled portabella mushroom (about five to six net carbs). Seafood lovers will appreciate the grilled salmon or shrimp (about two to three carbs). You can also get grilled chicken, pork chops, or ribs (leave off the BBQ sauce), all for zero carbs. Don't worry if you can't make up your mind—LongHorn offers combo meals so you can get two of your favorites. For side dishes, choose a small green salad or sliced tomatoes (about five net carbs each), steamed asparagus (about three net carbs), or other low-carb vegetables in season. LongHorn's tomato and onion salad combines thick, sliced, vine-ripe tomatoes layered with sliced red onion, crumbled bleu cheese, and balsamic vinaigrette dressing (about eight to ten net carbs). You can also get entrée-sized Caesar or garden salads with your choice of grilled steak, shrimp, chicken, or salmon (about ten to twelve net carbs without croutons).

MAGGIANO'S LITTLE ITALY
★★★★★ | $$$–$$$$$
www.maggianos.com
Nearly thirty restaurants in thirteen states and the
District of Columbia.
Claim to Fame: Italian cuisine

THE GOOD
Even though they don't specifically promote them,
Maggiano's menu offers a substantial number of no-
and low-carb menu choices—especially for an Italian
restaurant.

THE BAD
It's still Italian—of course there's going to be pasta and
lots of it. You'll also need to avoid one of Maggiano's
most popular side dishes, Vesuvio Roasted Potatoes,
served with garlic and olive oil.

THE UGLY
Maggiano's has a huge dessert menu with all your
classic Italian favorites, as well as nouvelle sweet
treats. Unfortunately, we low-carbers can't have
any of it.

The Best Things to Eat at Maggiano's Little Italy:
Maggiano's salad menu is particularly impressive, filled
with healthy low-carb meals with lots of satisfying,
flavorful ingredients. The salads here are really large, but
you can get a half-order. The approximate carb counts
listed below are for a large portion, enough to fill a
dinner plate.

Maggiano's salad combines iceberg and romaine lettuce,
crumbled blue cheese, crispy prosciutto, and red onions for
about four to six net carbs. You can get a chopped salad,
consisting of chopped iceberg lettuce, diced tomatoes,
crumbled blue cheese, green onion, avocado, and crispy

prosciutto, with or without chicken. Budget about eight to ten net carbs for the chopped salads, without croutons. At about fourteen and sixteen net carbs (without croutons or garbanzo beans), the Italian salad mixes iceberg and romaine lettuce with plum tomatoes, provolone cheese, broccoli, red onion, pepperocini, and roasted red peppers tossed with an Italian vinaigrette (if your diet encourages beans, keep the garbanzos in). Of course, you can also get a classic Caesar salad (hold the croutons, please) for about six to eight net carbs. When ordering entrées, remember you can always ask for them without sauce in order to keep the carb counts as low as possible, as in the following examples. For zero, or close to zero, carbs, order the prime bone-in rib eye, filet mignon, or the twelve or eighteen-ounce New York strip steaks, marinated in herbs and garlic, and broiled. Other no-carb protein entrées include the whole roast rosemary chicken, sautéed lemon herb salmon, or the garlic herb marinated veal chop. Side dishes at Maggiano's serve two or more. Order spinach, broccoli, or asparagus sautéed with garlic and olive oil for about three net carbs per half-cup serving.

MIMI'S CAFE
★★★ | $$–$$$
www.mimiscafe.com
Over eighty restaurants in nine states in the west, southwest, and south.
Claim to Fame: casual bistro fare

THE GOOD
Mimi's offers low-carbing customers a variety of full meals for just eight net carbs each. You'll also find a decent variety of low-carb lunches as well as breakfast, which is served all day long at Mimi's.

THE BAD
Beware of high-carb menu items like pasta, Mimi's famous chicken pot pie, or any number of breaded, fried things.

THE UGLY
In addition to the usual off-limits desserts, Mimi's serves a mighty tempting bread basket. Tell your server to take it away or, at minimum, sit as far away from its high-carb siren's call as possible.

The Best Things to Eat at Mimi's Cafe: For just eight net carbs, choose any of the following dinners, all served with steamed fresh vegetables: top sirloin or ribeye steak; savory pan-roasted chicken; blackened or broiled salmon and the fresh fish of the day. For lunch, try the petite cobb salad or a spinach, artichoke, and feta salad with balsamic vinaigrette (minus the usual croutons and sun-dried tomatoes), for just seven net carbs; the lettuce-wrapped Cafe Cheeseburger, served with cottage cheese, for eleven net carbs; or the chicken and vegetable platter, which also includes a green salad, for thirteen net carbs.

All of Mimi's low-carb breakfasts come with a glass of tomato juice and a side order of cottage cheese or fresh sliced tomatoes, included in the following net carb counts: the two-egg breakfast with bacon weighs in at eleven net carbs, twelve for eggs and sausage. For thirteen net carbs you can get a ham, broccoli, and cheddar omelet or Mimi's Low-Carb Breakfast, consisting of scrambled egg whites and an eight-ounce ground turkey patty.

ON THE BORDER MEXICAN GRILL & CANTINA

★★★★ | $$–$$$

www.ontheborder.com

Over 130 restaurants in thirty-one states.

Claim to Fame: Mexican food

THE GOOD

Guests can substitute low-carb sautéed vegetables for traditional Mexican rice and beans with all entrées here. While the restaurant is testing the possibility of low-carb tortillas, as of this writing they are still not available. Keep checking their Web site for menu changes.

THE BAD

This is Mexican food, so many menu items come wrapped in tortillas. All the appetizer items have some high-carb ingredients that render them unacceptable. All salads come with tortilla strips—lower the carb count by about ten grams by asking to have them omitted.

THE UGLY

This restaurant offers some creative south-of-the-border desserts. Unfortunately, low-carbers can't indulge.

The Best Things to Eat at On the Border Mexican Grill & Cantina: Take a gander at the fajita menu. As long as you have the discipline to forego the tortillas, there are lots of grilled meat and vegetable choices here—steak, chicken, shrimp, carnitas (pork), and portobello mushrooms. Other great entrée choices include the Grilled Salmon Mexicano (mesquite-grilled salmon served with mixed vegetables), Mexican Shrimp Scampi (shrimp sautéed in garlic and lime sauce), Pico Chicken and Shrimp (mesquite-grilled chicken topped with pico de gallo, garlic cilantro sauce, and Jack cheese, accompanied by four large sautéed shrimp), or Durango Steak and Shrimp (mesquite-grilled steak topped with Jack cheese, sautéed onions, poblano peppers, chile pepper sauce, and four large sautéed shrimp). None of these entrées should run over ten grams net carbs and most of those carbs are coming from healthy vegetables. For entrée salads, try the sizzling fajita salad (mixed greens, tomatoes, guacamole, sour cream, pico de gallo, and cheese with mesquite-grilled steak or chicken), or the chicken chopped salad (mixed greens with cheddar cheese, bacon, tomatoes, avocado, and grilled chicken). As long as you skip the tortilla strips, these salads should run about twelve to fourteen net carbs. You can also get a small side salad of mixed greens, tomatoes, and cheese to go with any entrée (about six net carbs).

OUTBACK STEAKHOUSE
★★★★ | $$–$$$

www.outbacksteakhouse.com
Hundreds of restaurants across the United States.
Claim to Fame: steaks and casual food served in
an Australian atmosphere

THE GOOD
An Aussie-style steakhouse would have to have a good
low-carb menu and Outback doesn't disappoint, with
all of your favorite cuts of beef along with grilled
chicken and fish. Low-carbers on road trips can use
the Outback Web site to plan meal stops at various
restaurants along the way.

THE BAD
Forget about the batter-fried Bloomin' Onion or the
Gold Coast Coconut Shrimp, which are breaded and
served with marmalade sauce. Ditto for other high-
carb and starchy items.

THE UGLY
Ignore Outback's specialty drink and dessert menus;
they will only tempt you with things you may desire,
but shouldn't have.

The Best Things to Eat at Outback Steakhouse:
Kookaburra (aka buffalo) wings are the only low-carb
appetizer Outback offers. No-carb entrée choices include
a wide variety of steaks, prime rib, rack of lamb (to keep
the carbs at zero, skip the cabernet sauce), grilled fish of
the day, grilled chicken breast (tell your server no BBQ
sauce, please), grilled salmon, or center-cut pork chops.
Accompany your entrée selection with a small green or
Caesar salad and steamed veggies. For an extra fee you
can get a side order of grilled shrimp and, for about
three carb grams, an order of sautéed mushrooms. For

about ten to twelve carbs (without croutons) order the meal-sized Brisbane Caesar salad, with or without grilled chicken or shrimp. For about thirteen to fifteen net carbs, the Steakhouse salad (minus the usual cinnamon pecans and Aussie chips) combines a seared sirloin steak atop a bed of mixed greens with tomatoes, red onions, and mushrooms.

RAINFOREST CAFÉ
★★★ | $$–$$$

www.rainforestcafe.com

Over thirty restaurants in sixteen states and five countries, mostly in large metropolitan and vacation areas.

Claim to Fame: casual food served in a tropical, rainforest-themed restaurant

THE GOOD

With its audio-animatronic animals and in-restaurant thunder storms, Rainforest Café is a place the whole family will love to visit. More importantly, low-carbing dieters will find plenty to eat while the kids are being amused and everyone is educated about the fragile rainforest ecosystem and what we can do to help.

THE BAD

Unquestionably, there are enough low-carb choices to make dining here interesting from a culinary perspective. That said, avoid anything on or in tortillas or bread, starchy appetizers, and sides such as fries or batter-fried foods and all pizzas and pastas.

THE UGLY

As usual, forget about desserts and avoid Rainforest Café's sweet signature cocktails.

The Best Things to Eat at Rainforest Café: Begin your meal with a Tsunami Shrimp Cocktail for about six net carbs per two tablespoons of sauce, or the Raging Thunder Buffalo Wings with celery, carrot sticks, and blue cheese dressing for about three to four net carb grams (about four net carbs per half-cup of carrots). Salad lovers will enjoy the Volcanic Cobb salad, or the Paradise house salad—a mixture of greens and Roma tomatoes, jicama, carrots, and cucumbers—for about eight to ten net carbs each. You can also get a meal-sized Caesar or grilled chicken Caesar salad (about six to eight net carbs without croutons) or a smaller Caesar that's perfect for a low-carb side dish, for about three to four net carbs. For zero carbs, try the Primal Steak, a fourteen-ounce New York Strip Steak, or the Tree Top Filet, a nine-ounce charbroiled tenderloin steak. Ask for steamed vegetables instead of the potatoes that usually come with entrées. In addition, you can find lots of great burgers at Rainforest Cafe; just be sure to order them without the bun.

RED LOBSTER

★★★★★ | $$–$$$$

www.redlobster.com

Over 650 restaurants forty-four states and four Canadian provinces.

Claim to Fame: seafood

THE GOOD

Low-carbing seafood lovers and landlubbers alike will find a dazzling array of menu choices at Red Lobster including broiled, grilled, and steamed fish and shellfish, juicy steaks, chicken, and salads.

THE BAD

Stay away from anything breaded and fried.

THE UGLY

The desserts at Red Lobster will sabotage your diet, but it's not hard to resist—there are so many good legal foods to eat here.

The Best Things to Eat at Red Lobster: The seafood choices at Red Lobster go on forever. Choose broiled, grilled, or blackened fish like salmon, trout, catfish or grouper, grilled mahi-mahi or Alaskan halibut, or broiled flounder—all for zero carbs. In the shellfish department, you can start your meal with a jumbo shrimp cocktail (about four carb grams in the sauce, zero for the shrimp); steamed or raw oysters on the half-shell (zero carbs without sauce); or steamed Prince Edward Island mussels (about four grams). Follow up with a steamed Maine lobster or Australian lobster tail, steamed snow crab legs, or broiled scallops, for zero carbs; or shrimp scampi, for about six carbs. If you're not into seafood, Red Lobster has a respectable selection of U.S.D.A. choice steaks, as well as grilled chicken dishes (zero carbs for the entrées). Having a hard time choosing? No problem. Red Lobster offers extensive combo dinners that let you have some of all your low-carb favorites. For side dishes, choose a small green or Caesar salad (no croutons, please) and steamed or grilled vegetables, for about four net carbs each.

RED ROBIN
★★★ | $$–$$$
www.redrobin.com
More than 200 restaurants in twenty-seven states and Canada.
Claim to Fame: gourmet burgers

THE GOOD
Toss the bread and you'll get some mighty good low-carb burgers at Red Robin.

THE BAD
Other than salads and breadless sandwiches, the other choices are bleak—all other entrées are battered, fried, or are otherwise prepared in a high-carb manner.

THE UGLY
If killer desserts weren't bad enough, Red Robin also offers monster shakes and malts and a bar full of sweet specialty drinks that will break the carb bank.

The Best Things to Eat at Red Robin: Red Robin's Buzzard Wings (aka buffalo wings) are the only low-carb appetizer, but at less than a gram for four wings, they're a good one. The Cobb salad makes a nice entrée, for about thirteen to fifteen net carbs. Otherwise, look to the burger menu. Red Robin offers twenty-two gourmet burgers. Keep yours no- or low-carb by choosing low-carb toppings like cheese, bacon, fried egg, sautéed mushrooms, lettuce, tomatoes, and onions. Avoid carb-laden condiments like BBQ or teriyaki sauce.

ROMANO'S MACARONI GRILL

★★★★★ | $$–$$$$

www.macaronigrill.com

Over 200 restaurants in thirty-eight states and five countries.

Claim to Fame: wood-fired pizza, pasta, and grilled food

THE GOOD

You'll find lots of great low-carb entrées and creative salads at this chain, but the best part is they have some unique side dishes that can really add variety to your diet. We especially liked the spinach sautéed with garlic, pecorino cheese, and lemon.

THE BAD

If you're a pizza, pasta, or bread fan, there's a lot of temptation to resist here. They make awesome wood-fired pizzas and calzonettos and, with a name like Macaroni Grill, the menu heavily features pasta.

THE UGLY

Macaroni Grill has a decadent dessert menu that even allows you to sample not one, not two, but three carb-laden dessert offerings. Don't even think about it.

The Best Things to Eat at Romano's Macaroni Grill: Macaroni Grill lets you skip the potatoes or pasta that normally accompany entrées and substitute sautéed spinach, Tuscan green beans, or grilled asparagus (about four net carbs each) or grilled tomatoes (about six to eight net carbs). Try the grilled salmon (ask your server to leave off the usual honey-teriyaki glaze), grilled pork chops, Pollo Magro, or "skinny chicken" (again, omit the honey balsamic glaze on these last two), or Tuscany ribeye, for zero carbs, not counting side dishes. For a handful of carbs, you can also order the chicken portobello. Consider starting your meal with Mozzarella alla Caprese—imported buffalo mozzarella, vine-ripened tomatoes, basil, and balsamic vinaigrette, for about eight to ten net carbs, or the Insalata Blu—Bibb lettuce, walnuts, red onions, blue cheese, and balsamic vinaigrette, for about six to eight net carbs. For about three net carbs, you can get a side Caesar salad (without croutons). The grilled tenderloin salad—beef tenderloin on baby arugula, spinach, radicchio, bacon, and blue cheese, with creamy Italian dressing is another carb bargain, but be sure to ask the kitchen to leave off the balsamic honey glaze that normally comes on it—about eight to ten net carbs.

RUBY TUESDAY
★★★★★ | $–$$$$
www.rubytuesday.com
Over 700 restaurants in forty states, Puerto Rico, and thirteen countries.
Claim to Fame: casual American food and drink

THE GOOD
Ruby Tuesday is the first restaurant of its kind to print nutritional data about every menu item right where you need it—on the actual menu itself. It doesn't get any easier or more convenient than that, folks. Or more frustrating; Ruby takes away every last excuse for cheating. That said, it's easy not to cheat here as you'll find over thirty low-carb menu options including (gasp!) a low-carb cheesecake for dessert. Keep in mind that Ruby Tuesday's menu changes frequently, so depending on when and where you visit, the exact items recommended below may or may not be available.

THE BAD
Even though there are lots of low-carb choices, this menu has about three times as many off-limit items—read the menu carefully and choose wisely.

THE UGLY
The dessert menu here is pretty tempting, but with a low-carb cheesecake offered, you won't feel the least bit deprived passing on the more decadent offerings. But just in case you're thinking about falling off the wagon, keep in mind that a slice of Ruby's Chocolate Tallcake contains 106 grams of carbohydrates.

The Best Things to Eat at Ruby Tuesday: For just one net carb per serving, start your meal with Veggies and Dip (broccoli, cherry tomatoes, red and green peppers, snap peas, and celery); a low-carb chicken quesadilla served in a high-fiber, whole wheat tortilla; or spicy buffalo wings served with blue cheese dressing and celery sticks. A bowl of hot broccoli cheese soup contains just nine net carb grams.

Reflected in the following carbs counts are the steamed broccoli and mashed cauliflower—a clever veggie that satisfies the mashed potato urge—that accompanies most entrées. Try the low-carb versions of Ruby's Church Street Chicken, grilled chicken with sautéed garlic mushrooms, bacon, and melted Swiss cheese, for zero carbs; Creole Catch (Cajun-seasoned, broiled tilapia), or chopped steak for one net carb each; New Orleans seafood (broiled tilapia topped with garlic shrimp and Alfredo sauce), or fresh baked turkey dinner with gravy, for four net carbs each. The veggie platter contains six net carb grams and the Peppercorn Chilean salmon has eight net carbs. Ruby's also offers a wide selection of steaks, none of which run over four net carbs per meal. You might also choose a chicken Caesar or spring chicken salad, for four net carbs each, or a turkey salad, for seven net carbs. For side dishes, you can get sautéed zucchini for one net carb; steamed broccoli for three; sugar snap peas or a spring mix salad for four net carbs; creamy mashed cauliflower for five; or creamed spinach for nine. In addition, you can construct your own perfect salad from Ruby's extensive salad bar.

Sandwich lovers can rejoice as Ruby Tuesday's offers a variety of low-carb wraps, served on whole-wheat tortillas. Try the burger wrap, turkey burger, or turkey burger club wraps, for two net carbs each; the Black and Blue wrap (peppercorn-seasoned burger topped with blue cheese, lettuce, tomatoes, and Dijon sauce) or peppercorn Jack wrap, for three net carbs; the spicy chicken wrap, for four; the peppercorn chicken wrap, for five; or the turkey wrap, for ten net carbs. Cap off your meal in a sweet way with a piece of low-carb cheesecake for just four net carbs. Finally—dessert is back!

SMOKEY BONES BBQ
★★★★ | $$$
www.smokeybones.com
Over seventy restaurants in seventeen states east
of the Mississippi.
Claim to Fame: BBQ ribs and meats

THE GOOD
Great steaks, pulled pork, grilled chicken, salmon,
and even buffalo burger served in a rustic mountain
lodge atmosphere give low-carbers lots of quality
protein options. In case you're into sports (or just
don't want to converse with your dinner companions), televisions fill the restaurant and each table
has its own volume control so you can choose to
watch or not.

THE BAD
Anything with BBQ sauce on it has too much sugar.
Monitor your side dishes, too—no baked beans,
beer-battered onion rings, potatoes, cole slaw, or
cinnamon apples.

THE UGLY
There are some delicious high-carb temptations lurking on the Smokey Bones menu, such as a cornbread
skillet with crushed pecan butter, bacon and cheese
potato slabs, chocolate fudge cake, or a bag of freshly
made cinnamon sugar donuts. Ouch!

The Best Things to Eat at Smokey Bones BBQ: Buffalo
wings served with celery sticks and blue cheese dressing
provide a tasty carb-free appetizer. While the ribs here
are basted with sauce during cooking, Smokey Bones's
smoked tender pulled pork isn't, making it a satisfying
no-carb entrée—providing you can resist slathering it in
BBQ sauce once it arrives at the table. You'll also find a

variety of steaks available for zero carbs, as well as grilled Atlantic salmon and balsamic marinated grilled chicken breasts. For an extra fee, you can add a grilled chicken breast or shrimp skewer to any entrée. For side dishes, choose green beans, steamed broccoli, or, when in season, steamed asparagus, for about three net carbs each, and/or a small green salad, for about six net carbs. For about ten to twelve net carbs, consider the Cobb salad. If you want something a little out of the ordinary, don't miss Smokey Bones's buffalo burger (bunless, of course).

STEAK & ALE
★★★★★ | $$$–$$$$$
www.steakandale.com

Over sixty restaurants mostly in the east, south,
and midwest.
Claim to Fame: steaks

THE GOOD
You'll find lots to eat at Steak and Ale besides
great steaks, including seafood, chicken, salads, and
veggies. This chain is well aware of low-carbers and
has special side dishes and menu combinations that
cater to them.

THE BAD
Beware of the usual suspects—baked and fried potatoes,
pastas, starchy appetizers, and sweet BBQ sauces.

THE UGLY
The Cheesy Garlic Loaf is a tempting freshly baked
loaf of bread brushed with garlic butter and topped
with melted cheese. Steak and Ale also offers a
respectable collection of decadent desserts. Don't go
anywhere near these carbohydrate repositories.

The Best Things to Eat at Steak & Ale: Look no further
than Steak & Ale's carb-counter lunch and dinner menus.
All entrées (except the sirloin salad) come with low-carb
steamed veggies (reflected in the carb counts below).

At dinnertime, you can dine on the mushroom stuffed
filet (six or nine ounces) or the surf and turf dinners (a
six-ounce filet and shrimp scampi), for just nine carb
grams each. For ten carbs, try the filet of Alaskan rock sole
brushed with garlic butter, served with shrimp scampi, or
the lemon-herb marinated shrimp skewers. For fourteen
grams, the grilled sirloin salad gives you a seven-ounce

sirloin steak sliced over mixed greens with tomatoes, crumbled bacon, and mushrooms topped with blue cheese dressing.

At lunchtime, in addition to the Alaskan rock sole and sirloin salad, you can also get the smoked cheddar burger au naturel, a half-pound burger topped with melted smoked cheddar cheese, lettuce, tomato, and onion; or the grilled chicken sandwich au naturel (grilled chicken breast with provolone cheese, bacon, lettuce, tomato, and onion), for just seven carb grams. For nine grams, order the blue burger au naturel, a half-pound burger topped with crumbled blue cheese, blue cheese dressing, bacon, lettuce, tomato, and onion.

STUART ANDERSON'S BLACK ANGUS
★★★★★ | $$$–$$$$$

www.stuartandersons.com

Over 100 restaurants in twelve states, with concentrations in the west.

Claim to Fame: steaks

THE GOOD

Stuart Anderson's Black Angus offers a large variety of no- and low-carb entrées—steaks, prime ribs, chicken, fish, and shellfish—so whatever you're in the mood for, you're likely to find it. Their bottomless garden salad side dish is a nice touch, too.

THE BAD

Low-carb side dishes are limited to a steamed vegetable medley and green salad. It would be nice to have a few other veggie choices. Pass on the sandwiches and burgers and go to the protein entrées or salads. Of course, skip the usual high-carb bombs like potatoes, bread, and anything breaded and fried.

THE UGLY

The dessert menu is a killer. Trust me, don't even sneak a peek.

The Best Things to Eat at Stuart Anderson's Black Angus: Begin your meal with a shrimp cocktail (about six net carbs in the cocktail sauce, so eat less sauce and ingest less carbs) or an order of hot wings, for less than one carb per six wings. You'll find a chuckwagon full of entrée options at this western-style steakhouse. Beef lovers will enjoy the filet mignon, New York, T-bone, ribeye, and top sirloin steaks, all for zero carbs. Dress up a filet mignon with blue cheese and mushrooms for fewer than three net carbs. You can also get prime rib in three cuts—half-pound, three quarters of a pound, or a full pound. Trying to eat less red meat? Try the grilled lemon pepper chicken, garlic spiced scallops, or lemon garlic grilled prawns (about one carb each), baked salmon, steamed lobster tail, or grilled ahi tuna (zero carbs as long as you pass on the pineapple salsa that normally comes with the ahi). Don't worry if you can't decide; Black Angus offers several combo dinners and, for an extra charge, you can add a petite lobster tail, grilled shrimp, or scallops to any entrée.

For side dishes, choose steamed mixed vegetables and a bottomless garden salad with low-carb dressing like blue cheese or oil and vinegar. You can also get entrée-sized Cobb and chicken Caesar salads; neither should run over 10 carb grams providing you skip the croutons.

TEXAS ROADHOUSE
★★★★ | $$–$$$

www.texasroadhouse.com
Over 150 restaurants in thirty-two states.
Claim to Fame: steaks and ribs

THE GOOD
Great steaks, prime rib, roasted chicken, grilled salmon, and more—the Roadhouse serves up lots of low-carb options.

THE BAD
There are lots of breaded and high-carb items, too, especially on the appetizer menu and among the side dishes. The BBQ sauce that normally comes on this restaurant's award-winning ribs is high in sugar, but you can ask to have it omitted.

THE UGLY
Baked potatoes and sweet potatoes loaded with marshmallows and caramel sauce will definitely break the carb bank, as will the desserts (luckily there aren't too many of these).

The Best Things to Eat at Texas Roadhouse: For zero carbs, it's hard to beat any of Texas Roadhouse's steaks, oven-roasted chicken, or grilled salmon. The ribs also qualify, providing you ask your server to leave the BBQ sauce off. Can't decide? Texas Roadhouse also offers combo meals that give you some of each. Instead of high-carb sides, order the green beans (about three net carbs), steamed vegetable medley (about five net carbs), or a small green or Caesar salad (without croutons) for about three net carbs. Start your meal with an order of "naked" (unbreaded) buffalo wings, for an almost carb-free appetizer. Salad lovers can order the grilled chicken salad (about ten net carbs) or chicken Caesar salad (about six net carbs without croutons).

T.G.I. FRIDAY'S
★★★★ | $$–$$$$

www.tgifridays.com

Five hundred and twenty-seven in forty-seven states; two hundred and eight in five countries.
Claim to Fame: casual American food and drink

THE GOOD

In addition to the low-carb options on their regular menu, T.G.I. Friday's offers an Atkins-approved menu of certified low-carb offerings.

THE BAD

As usual, the regular appetizer menu is off limits, with the exception of buffalo wings, the perennial low-carb favorite. If you venture off the Atkins menu, order carefully. The regular menu at T.G.I. Friday's is peppered with lots of breaded fried things, food served in or on some sort of bread, rice, or pasta, and often slathered in some sort of sweet sauce or glaze.

THE UGLY

T.G.I. Friday's is known for their drinks; they even sponsor competitions for their bartenders. There are lots of fabulous sweet, high-carb cocktails—some even have ice cream and suspiciously resemble milkshakes. Stick to the food here, or, if you must drink, keep it simple. That means light beers, a glass of wine, or a no-carb cocktail like rum and diet cola.

The Best Things to Eat at TGI Friday's: You can't go wrong ordering from the Atkins menu as all the low-carb choices are already made for you. Start your meal with some buffalo wings for five net carbs. Or share an order of Tuscan spinach dip served with fresh vegetables. The total order contains seventeen net carbs; however, it's doubtful one person could eat the entire rich dish (a blend of parmesan and romano cheeses blended with spinach, artichokes, sautéed onions, and peppers) themselves, even if they were very hungry. For just six net carbs you can order the char-grilled salmon filet, topped with capers and lemon sauce; the New York strip steak topped with blue cheese and served with steamed broccoli; or a double bunless burger topped with melted cheese and served with mixed greens. Seven net carbs buys you a plate of garlic chicken served with a mix of sautéed Roma tomatoes, red peppers, zucchini, and squash. An Atkins-friendly grilled chicken Caesar salad weighs in at nine net carbs. The most unique low-carb dish served is the tuna salad wrap, made with white Albacore, water chestnuts, and a hint of wasabi, served with a side of pineapple. The dish serves up fourteen net carbs, but you can skip the pineapple and lower that number to ten. T.G.I.'s sizzling chicken with broccoli is typically served with onions and peppers and melted cheese, for seventeen net carbs. You can shave five carbs from that total by skipping the onions and peppers.

TONY ROMA'S
★★★★ | $$–$$$
www.tonyromas.com
Over two hundred and sixty restaurants across the
United States and in twenty-seven countries.
Claim to Fame: ribs

THE GOOD
Tony Roma's new Nada-Carb BBQ Sauce has zero
grams net carbs, opening up a world of previously
off-limits BBQ meals for low-carbs dieters.

THE BAD
Don't slip and order the regular BBQ sauces as they
can easily add fifteen to twenty carb grams or more
to your daily total.

THE UGLY
As usual, stay away from the dessert menu, potatoes,
and bread.

The Best Things to Eat at Tony Roma's: Tony Roma's
is known for ribs, but they also offer a variety of steaks,
grilled chicken, and salmon. To keep any of these entrées
at zero net carbs (except the baby back ribs, which have
one gram), be sure to order it with Tony's new Nada-
Carb BBQ sauce. Pair your dinner or lunch with steamed
broccoli (three net carbs) and a low-carb house salad (six
net carbs). Wash down your meal with an ice-cold bottle
of Coor's Aspen Edge beer, for just 2.6 carbs.

Upscale Restaurants

BENIHANA
★★★ | $$$$–$$$$$
www.benihana.com

Over seventy restaurants across the United States and in South America, Europe, Asia, and Australia.
Claim to Fame: Japanese teppan cuisine prepared tableside in a highly entertaining manner.

THE GOOD
An evening at Benihana is more than just a meal; it's a culinary show, with skilled chefs slicing, dicing, and flipping food, dramatically preparing dishes right before your eyes. It's a lot of fun, and low-carbers will find lots of tasty things to eat here, as long as they pass on the rice and noodles. Everything here is cooked to order right in front of you, so it's easy to make special requests.

THE BAD
Benihana also serves sushi, which you'll need to avoid because of the rice. Rice or noodles accompany every menu item. Don't eat them. Avoid the Yakisoba, or stir-fried noodle, dinner. The Seafood Diablo also comes with noodles. Don't order anything with teriyaki sauce, as it's loaded with sugar.

THE UGLY
Meals come with dessert, fruit, or a cup of ice cream. Tell your server to leave yours in the kitchen or immediately give it to a dinner companion.

The Best Things to Eat at Benihana: If you follow the rules—no rice, nothing served with noodles or teriyaki sauce—the rest of the Teppanyaki menu is pretty much in play. Choose from Hibachi chicken, steak, shrimp, scallops, or lobster, for zero carbs, all served with a no-carb appetizer of grilled shrimp and a carb-legal mix of hibachi vegetables. The cup of soup that comes with the meal should run no more than eight to ten carbs. Ask for salad dressing on the side; Benihana's dressing has a little sugar in it—not enough to make a noticeable dent in your daily carb budget, but do try to use as little as possible.

HOUSTON'S

★★★★ | $$$–$$$$$

www.houstons.com

Currently thirty-nine restaurants in major metropolitan areas in thirteen states.

Claim to Fame: upscale American food

THE GOOD

There are lots of terrific protein choices at Houston's, along with vegetable side dishes that highlight the best of seasonal produce.

THE BAD

Houston's grilled chicken salad—a good low-carb choice in most restaurants—is augmented by tortilla strips, peanut sauce, and a honey-lime vinaigrette dressing. Realize that if you order this, you'll have to do some major revamping to keep the carb count acceptable.

THE UGLY

Beware of the diet-busting hand-cut French fries, cheddar parmesan toast, five-nut brownie, or apple walnut cobbler. Let's not even talk about the damage a loaded baked potato could do.

The Best Things to Eat at Houston's: You can get steamed vegetables with any of Houston's entrées instead of the usual high-carb fare; choices will change daily based on the best the market has to offer. If your diet allows grains, you can order side dishes of brown rice and black beans or couscous.

Vegetables and fish choices change with the season and market availability, but you will always find a seafood of the day at Houston's that can be grilled for zero carbs. Other virtually carb-free entrées include rotisserie chicken, seared ahi tuna, prime rib roast, double cut pork chops, or filet mignon. For an extra fee, you can get a small Houston's salad or Caesar salad (about four to six net carbs each without dressing or croutons). Also available are entrée versions of these salads, for about twelve to fifteen grams. While others at your table indulge in dessert, finish your meal with an espresso or cappuccino and no-carb sweetener.

MCCORMICK & SCHMICK'S
★★★★★ | $$$–$$$$

www.mccormickandschmicks.com
Over forty-five restaurants in major metropolitan
areas in twenty states.
Claim to Fame: seafood

THE GOOD
The best seafood and produce available at the market on any particular day determines the menu at
McCormick & Schmick's. These people know how
to put it together. They print a new menu each day
and every day, featuring between 85 and 110 dishes.
Low-carbers can always count on getting a huge
selection of fish and shellfish here, along with more
traditional fare like steaks and poultry.

THE BAD
Stay away from pastas, baked potatoes, rice, and anything that's breaded and fried. The menu here is so
huge it's easy to avoid the no-no's.

THE UGLY
Of course, there's an off-limits dessert menu.
McCormick & Schmick's also makes some awesome
cocktails the old-fashioned way, with fresh-squeezed,
real fruit juice and mixers. Unfortunately, most are
high in carbs. If you must drink, stick to light beer, a
glass of wine, or a no-carb drink such as scotch and
soda or whiskey and diet cola.

The Best Things to Eat at McCormick & Schmick's:
Since the menu changes daily, it's impossible to make
exact recommendations for this restaurant, but feel confident you'll find a lot to eat at M&S. Stick to the low-
carb rules. As you've been reading this book, you'll have
noticed a pattern: grilled, broiled, blackened, or steamed

are okay; breaded and fried is not. Pair your preferred cooking method with your favorite fish from the daily selection. You can also get terrific shellfish like shrimp, scallops, crab, and lobster. For side dishes, order steamed vegetables—again, the market dictates what's served on any given day—and a green salad. You could easily make a meal of the appetizer menu by ordering items like raw and steamed oysters, steamed shrimp, and clams. If you're not into seafood, don't worry. You'll also find a nice selection of meat and poultry dishes here.

Be sure to check out Happy Hour at McCormick & Schmick's, especially if you're on a budget. The ultra-low priced bar menu changes daily, but almost always contains a few items that low-carbers can eat—oyster shooters, peel-and-eat shrimp, or bunless burgers. Stick to no-carb drinks like light beer, red wine, or rum and diet cola, or something nonalcoholic and non-carb. One more important note: M&S's doesn't stick to conventional happy hours. The phenomenal food bargains offered are designed to attract customers to the bar during otherwise slow periods. The exact happy hours vary at each individual McCormick & Schmick's, so call the restaurant you plan to visit for exact details. Most stores offer a late afternoon happy hour; for example, three to six P.M., some restaurants offer another happy hour session in the late evening; for instance, 9:30 until closing. Still others offer an all-day Sunday happy hour. But, in all cases, when other bars typically celebrate Happy Hour, McCormick & Schmick's is full price.

MORTON'S: THE STEAKHOUSE
★★★★★ | $$$$$

www.mortons.com

Over sixty restaurants in major metropolitan areas in twenty-eight states and four countries.

Claim to Fame: steaks

THE GOOD

There's something for the low-carber in every part of Morton's menu, from appetizers to desserts. A fabulous special occasion restaurant, the food and service at Morton's are first-rate and the menu is overflowing with excellent no- and low-carb choices.

THE BAD

Morton's is one of the rare restaurants whose menu is more good than bad from a low-carb perspective. Just make sure you don't eat potatoes in any of the five wonderful ways that Morton's prepares them.

THE UGLY

The dessert menu here is to die for (as in the death of your diet)—Godiva cake, hot upside-down apple pie, and soufflés—to name a few. Fill up on all the great legal foods Morton's has to offer so you won't be tempted.

The Best Things to Eat at Morton's: Start your dining experience with a no-carb appetizer: colossal shrimp cocktail, bluepoint oysters on the half shell, smoked pacific salmon, jumbo lump crabmeat cocktail, or broiled sea scallops wrapped in bacon. Skip the apricot chutney that normally comes with the scallops and add two and six carb grams, depending on how much cocktail sauce you consume. For entrées, have fun choosing between the various cuts of Morton's steaks, veal chops, lamb chops, broiled salmon fillet, whole baked Maine lobster, and, when available, prime rib. The sauces like *beurre blanc* or *béarnaise* that accompany some of the entrées have minimal carbs, about four grams per two tablespoons. Morton's really shines in the side dish department, an area where most other restaurants lack. Try a spinach, Caesar, or Morton's house salad (about six net carbs without croutons or dressing), or, for something different, try the sliced beefsteak tomato, purple onion and blue cheese salad, for about eight to ten net carbs. For vegetables, you can get fresh steamed asparagus (about seven to eight net carbs) or broccoli (about seven net carbs), with or without hollandaise sauce (about four carbs per two tablespoons), sautéed fresh spinach and mushrooms (about seven to ten net carbs), sautéed wild mushrooms with sautéed onions (about eight to ten net carbs), and creamed spinach (about ten net carbs per half-cup). Finish your meal with a nice espresso or cappuccino. If your diet plan allows it, Morton's dessert menu usually includes fresh seasonal berries. Skip the tasty but sweet sabayon sauce that usually adorns the berries and eat them plain or with a little whipped cream instead. Berries have the lowest carb counts of all the fruits. According to the U.S.D.A. food database, a cup of blackberries contains 6.4 net carbs, 6.69 for raspberries, 8.16 for strawberries, and 17.51 for blueberries.

P. F. CHANG'S CHINA BISTRO
★★★ | $$$–$$$$
www.pfchangs.com
Over 100 restaurants in thirty states.
Claim to Fame: Chinese cuisine

THE GOOD
P.F. Chang's new Training Table menu, designed in conjunction with the restaurant's sponsorship of the P. F. Chang's Rock 'n' Roll Arizona Marathon and Half Marathon, gives low-carb dieters a respectable number of choices in the usually bleak, carb-laden landscape of Chinese cuisine.

THE BAD
Many menu items are high-carb in and of themselves, before being paired with rice or noodles.

THE UGLY
Some dishes that may seem like they should be low in carbs actually aren't, due to sauces and thickening agents. For instance, a full order of chicken lettuce wraps packs in ninety-seven carb grams; ninety-one grams for garlic sugar snap peas. There are tons of tempting high-carb rice and noodle dishes on the P. F. Chang's menu, not to mention desserts that include a six-layer chocolate cake and banana spring rolls.

The Best Things to Eat at P. F. Chang's: If some of the carb counts below seem higher than most of the recommendations in this book it's because the number represents the total number of carbs in the entire dish, which is usually enough to share with a friend or two. Divide the carbs according to how much of the dish you actually consume.

Begin your meal with an appetizer of northern style spare ribs, for just six carb grams, or seared ahi tuna rolled in Chinese spices and served cold with spicy mustard on a bed of soybean sprouts and pea shoots, for fifteen carbs. For entrées try P. F. Chang's steamed salmon (five carbs), Cantonese shrimp (eight), Cantonese scallops (fifteen), chicken with black bean sauce, or Moo Goo Gai Pan (nineteen). Low-carb side dishes include Shanghai cucumbers, for about five net carbs, garlic spinach for fifteen, or Sichuan asparagus for thirty-four.

RUTH'S CHRIS STEAK HOUSE
★★★★★ | $$$$$
www.ruthschris.com
Over seventy restaurants in twenty-nine states and Canada.
Claim to Fame: steaks

THE GOOD
It doesn't get any better than this, friends. Ruth's Chris is the ultimate low-carb, special occasion restaurant. Everything about this upscale chain is world-class, from melt-in-your-mouth tender steaks to the extensive international wine list to the freshly made salad dressings. Everything is served à la carte, so you can order exactly what you want and avoid anything you don't, and Ruth's Chris has some truly fabulous low-carb side dishes to augment its legendary low steaks.

THE BAD
A few of the decadent starchy sides will be off limits. The bread basket could wreak major damage on your diet. Ask your server to take it away or try to sit on the other side of the table from this temptation.

THE UGLY
The desserts at Ruth's Chris are as good as its steaks, but low-carbers can't indulge. Luckily, the rest of the meal here is so spectacular, you won't miss them. Indulge in a nice espresso or cappuccino instead.

The Best Things to Eat at Ruth's Chris: Start your meal with a shrimp remoulade cocktail, for about four carb grams, or the virtually carb-free seared ahi tuna. Don't skip salad; Ruth's makes their own delicious dressings (the blue cheese can't be beat). Order the Steak House salad, Caesar salad, iceberg lettuce wedge, or Ruth's chopped salad, but save yourself ten to twelve carb grams and skip the croutons.

For no- and ultra-low-carb entrées, choose any of Ruth's signature steaks, broiled North Atlantic salmon, lamb chops, Maine lobster, Australian lobster tail, ahi tuna steak, or stuffed chicken breast—an oven-roasted double chicken breast stuffed with garlic herb cheese and served with lemon butter. Accompany your entrée with Fresh asparagus with Hollandaise sauce (about six net carbs), a broiled tomato (about five net carbs), or sautéed mushrooms (about three net carbs).